Coeliac Disease

Coeliac Disease

Nursing Care and Management

Helen Griffiths MSc, RGN, Cert MHSC

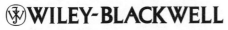

A John Wiley & Sons, Ltd., Publication

This edition first published 2008
© 2008 John Wiley & Sons

Wiley-Blackwell is an imprint of John Wiley & Sons, formed by the merger of Wiley's global
Scientific, Technical and Medical business with Blackwell Publishing.

Registered office
John Wiley & Sons Ltd, The Atrium, Southern Gate, Chichester, West Sussex, PO19 8SQ,
United Kingdom

Editorial office
John Wiley & Sons Ltd, The Atrium, Southern Gate, Chichester, West Sussex, PO19 8SQ,
United Kingdom

For details of our global editorial offices, for customer services and for information about
how to apply for permission to reuse the copyright material in this book please see our
website at www.wiley.com/wiley-blackwell.

Library of Congress Cataloging-in-Publication Data

Griffiths, Helen, 1962–
Coeliac disease : nursing care and management / Helen Griffiths.
    p. ; cm.
Includes bibliographical references and index.
ISBN 978-0-470-51260-9 (pbk.)
1. Coeliac disease – Nursing.   I. Title.
[DNLM: 1. Coeliac Disease.   2. Coeliac Disease – nursing. WD 175 G855c 2008]

RC862.C44G75 2008
616.3'99–dc22

                              2008019021

A catalogue record for this book is available from the British Library

Typeset in 10/12.5pt Palatino by Aptara Inc., New Delhi, India
Printed in Singapore by Markono Print Media Pte Ltd

1   2008

This book is dedicated to my father
whose belief
in me remains my beacon.
And my family who helps to keep it
blazing

Contents

List of Contributors

Elaine Horne BSc, RGN
Clinical Nurse Specialist Gastroenterology,
Hereford Hospitals NHS Trust

James Horne,
Student

Patient Stories:
Alan Holmes
Zoe Verry
Jean Lloyd

Foreword

Helen has brought together years of experience of managing coeliac disease in this highly informative new book. It provides an excellent source of information for Specialist Nurses developing an up-to-date service for patients with coeliac disease and will also be a valuable source of information for patients and their families in exploring the many issues of this condition. The extensive literature search and detailed medical discussions will be of great interest to general practitioners and hospital specialists as the full range of holistic care of patients with coeliac disease is addressed. The multitude of real-life experiences that come out of every chapter make this a living account of the impact of coeliac disease on patients' every day lives and how all healthcare professionals can work together for the patients' benefit.

The individual chapters address the different aspects of coeliac disease in a clear but thorough manner with the final chapter of four true life stories bringing the most important issues together in patients' own words. Each of the preceding chapters have learning outcomes clearly laid out and also activities to improve the development of health services with particular emphasis on the type of patient information that is useful and practical.

The crucial question of accurate diagnosis is addressed not only from the scientific perspective of serological screening tests but also from how to undertake the initial and probably most important first consultation in the most productive way possible. The issue of the coeliac iceberg is developed with the 'below the waterline' concept introduced. Dietary management is considered as a medical nutrition therapy with international standards of food labelling addressed in a thorough manner.

Practical advice of shopping lists for eating in is listed and good-humoured recommendations for eating out are given. The emotional impact of dealing with the diagnosis receives a rewarding amount of discussion and vulnerable groups in adolescence, pregnancy and old age are given specific consideration.

The team approach to the management of coeliac disease is considered essential with long-term aim of dietary compliance as the key to successful management. The option of telephone follow-up clinics is outlined but only if that is in the best interest of individual patients. The role of patient support groups and their benefits are discussed along with the issue of patient expectations.

Potential complications of osteoporosis, hyposplenism and risk of malignancy are carefully appraised with the evidence and current understanding of these complications described. Difficulties in management of resistant disease cover interesting possibilities of cross-contamination in addition to the rarer medical diagnoses of bacterial overgrowth, microscopic colitis and exocrine pancreatic insufficiency.

Future developments and current avenues of research are outlined with fascinating possibilities of dietary supplementation with endopeptidases, detoxification by transamidation of wheat flour and genetic modification of cereals to selectively reduce the toxic component of gluten.

This book has clearly been written to be enjoyed by a wide range of readers with the ultimate aim of improving the care and management of all patients with coeliac disease.

Dr Rupert A.J. Ransford, MRCGP, MD, FRCP
Consultant Gastroenterologist &
Clinical Director for Medicine
Hereford Hospitals
NHS Trust

Preface

It is thought that coeliac disease affects as many as 1:100 people in the United Kingdom, many of whom will remain undiagnosed.

The aim of this book is to provide nurses with the knowledge and understanding to not only help identify those possibly affected but understand the investigative pathway, the impact of the diagnosis and the long-term treatment and management.

The treatment of coeliac disease is the 'life-long' dietary exclusion of the protein gluten, found in wheat, barley, oats and rye. Anyone who has had their diet restricted voluntarily (weight watching) or involuntarily, even for a brief time, will know how attractive prohibited foods can be. Therefore, it should not be assumed that life-long dietary restriction is either easy or sustainable, but it is imperative if the long-term health risks associated with coeliac disease are to be avoided.

In my work as a nurse consultant and endoscopist I have come to appreciate the enormous impact that diagnosis and treatment can have on individuals with coeliac disease and the value of good support. This book is written to help nurses, through knowledge and understanding, and add value to the lives of those in their care with coeliac disease.

Introduction and How to Use This Book

'I read and I forget
I see and I remember
I do and I understand'
(Adapted from Confucius, 551–479 BC)

This quote will ring a salient bell with many of us; the busier we are, the less effectively we read and the less likely we are to remember what we have read unless it becomes a routine part of our lives. Hence, despite our best intentions when we sit down with a medical book meaning to enhance our knowledge on a subject, the chances are that we will skip bits or skim read and then still find ourselves a few weeks later saying 'I'm sure I read something about that'. Sound familiar?

The aim of this book is threefold:

- To increase nurses' knowledge and understanding of the care and management of coeliac disease.
- To enable general nurses to understand the health needs of coeliac patients in their care.
- To assist specialist nurses in developing services for coeliac patients.

To support these aims, each chapter has been designed to impart knowledge, but also to try and move you from simply reading to 'doing' something for coeliac patients and therefore understanding more fully the impact of this disease on individuals. In order to do this you will find a number of boxes within the text.

At the start of each chapter you will find a box with:

> **Intended learning outcomes, which will:**
> - Help you to make best use of each chapter
> - Maximise your knowledge intake
> - Help put theory into practice

The text is also interspersed with boxes highlighting:

> **Activities that will help you to:**
> Think about the information contained in each chapter and demonstrate how this might relate to and improve practice within your own clinical area.

In addition there are:

> **Hints and tips for service development:**
> With practical advice for nurses working within specialist areas who wish to provide dedicated supportive services for coeliac patients.

For specialist nurses hoping to develop a specific service for coeliac patients it is important to follow some basic principles which I hope you will find within this text:

- That the service is built on current evidence-based practice but remains responsive to growing evidence.
- That there are real benefits for patients including improved access to care at a time that is appropriate and timely and acknowledges coeliac disease as a long-term condition.
- That it is built around pathways and protocols that support the evidence base and audit its effectiveness.
- That links are maintained with all those involved in the service.
- That the personal and professional development and learning required in undertaking the role is acknowledged and built into the service.

Rather than detract from the readability of the text it is hoped that it will maximise your learning and lead to greater understanding.

Chapter 1
The History of Coeliac Disease

LEARNING OUTCOMES

At the end of this chapter you should be able to:

- Describe where the word 'coeliac' came from.
- Chart the early history of the disease.
- Critically discuss the current diagnostic criteria.

At the end of the last Ice Age, as we moved from the Mesolithic into the Neolithic era, people discovered that if they settled in one place for long enough, instead of relying on their hunter gatherer nomadic existence, they could sow and harvest crops of cereals like wheat.

One of the consequences of this Neolithic revolution was civilisation and the concept of production. Another, in all probability, was that people who could not tolerate wheat as part of their diet became ill.

We can surmise that coeliac disease has always existed. However, despite its first description as a clinical entity as far back as the second century AD, the fact that its numerous symptoms mimic several other conditions and that its cause has remained elusive has meant that its recognition as a distinct disorder, readily diagnosed and treated, has been a long and complicated journey. This is why history is so important, not only from the point of view of general interest but in helping both the healthcare profession and patients understand the complexity of the disease.

> **Activity**
>
> How do you think that the history of the disease might be useful when discussing the diagnosis with patients?
> Consider here how you would feel if your diagnosis had been made after many years of feeling 'unwell'. Could the fact that our understanding has been slow be reassuring?

This is written with the understanding that when we talk of 'history' in coeliac disease, as more is known about the disease and its management even recent findings become history.

We start this chapter by describing the history of the disease, the history that led to the recognition of the environmental factors triggering the disease and the notable medical contributions made to its recognition as a distinct disorder. We then look at its definition and the challenges to the diagnostic criteria.

A CHRONOLOGICAL HISTORY OF COELIAC DISEASE

The second century AD

The word coeliac comes from the Greek word *koiliakos*, meaning 'suffering in the bowels'. This was the term used by Aretaeus of Cappadocia, a contemporary of the Roman Physician Galen in the second half of the second century AD. From his writings, edited and translated from Greek to Latin by Francis Adams and printed for the Sydenham Society of England in 1856 (Adams, 1856), koiliakos first became known as 'The Coeliac Affection'. *An affection of the digestion and of the distribution.*

In these translations we find the first descriptions of the disease, with features including fatty diarrhoea, pallor, weight loss and chronic relapse, affecting both children and adults. Aretaeus described the diarrhoea as being light in colour, offensive in odour and accompanied by flatulence. The patient he described as emaciated and atrophied and incapable of performing any of his accustomed works.

The seventeenth century

Just a year prior to Adams' (1856) translation of Aretaeus' works, Dr Gull writing in Guy's hospital reports (Gull, 1855) outlined the case of a 13-year-old boy, whose symptoms of enlarged abdomen and frequent and voluminous stools of a dull, chalky colour clearly suggested the symptoms of coeliac disease as we understand them today. However, it was not until a few years later in 1888 that Dr Samuel Gee, using the same title as Francis Adams' (1856) translation, gave the second classic and first modern description of 'The Coeliac Affection' and laid the foundation not only for describing the condition, but also for establishing a criterion for its diagnosis and furthermore a recognition of its treatment being related to diet.

Gee (1888) described coeliac as a kind of chronic indigestion, affecting people of all ages but especially children between 1 and 5 years of age. As with Aretaeus, he describes a pale, loose, foul-smelling stool, frothy in appearance, resembling oatmeal porridge or gruel. He paints a vivid picture of a wasted almost cachectic patient, pale and puffy of face. He observes that unfortunately death is a common end and where patients survive, recovery is often incomplete, the illness dragging on for years with periods of relapse.

Dr Gee (1888) identified a causative link between the symptoms of emaciation, cachexia and diarrhoea and for the first time, rather prophetically, that (Gee, 1888):

> if the patient can be cured at all, it must be by means of diet (p. 20).

He made the observation that rice, sago and cornflour were unfit foods and that malted foods including rusks and bread were better. Although we now know the reverse to be true, for the first time Gee (1888) implied that unfit foods actually produced a pathologic condition of the digestive tract.

What the patient takes beyond his power of digestion does harm (p. 20).

The twentieth century

The next important breakthrough in our understanding of coeliac disease did not come until 1908, as a culmination of 7 years of work between Dr Emmett Holt, senior director of children's medicine at Bellevue Hospital, and Christian Herter of Columbia University. They worked together on both the clinical and theoretical aspects of the disease and published their conclusions in a work entitled *On Infantilism from Chronic Intestinal Infection* (Herter, 1908). Their main observations were that this was a pathological state of childhood associated with a chronic intestinal infection. The chief manifestations of this intestinal infantilism were an arrest in the development of the body, without affecting mental development. It was, however, characterised by marked abdominal distension, a varying degree of anaemia, rapid onset of physical and mental fatigue, and irregularities of intestinal digestion resulting in frequent episodes of diarrhoea. Their most important contribution was the observation that whilst fats were tolerated moderately well, carbohydrates were poorly tolerated, almost always causing relapse or a return of diarrhoea. Whilst these conclusions were not universally accepted by colleagues, they did act as the catalyst for further research into the most effective dietary treatment.

Two assistants of Dr Holt, Dr John Howland and Dr Sidney Haas, took up the cause of their senior colleagues and in 1921, Dr Howland in his presidential address to the American Paediatric Society (Newland, 1921) presented a paper on *Prolonged Intolerance to Carbohydrates*. He observed that growth suffered in proportion to the length of time that symptoms persisted and that many children were as a consequence below the average in height. He again noted that of all the elements of food, carbohydrate was the one that had to be most rigorously excluded and that after initial improvement in symptoms, was the most difficult to add back into the diet. He particularly noted that bread and cereals were the last foods that could be reintroduced to the diet. Unsurprisingly, Howland's treatment achieved greater success than previous diets, but the question remained as to whether carbohydrates could be tolerated at all?

So was it all bananas?

It was Howland's partner, Dr Sydney Haas, following on from Howland's work, who introduced the banana diet. He noted from reports published over the years that children with severe diarrhoea did well on banana flour and plantain meal. At the time bananas were considered to be completely indigestible by a sick child. However, his experiments at the Home for Hebrew Infants (Golden Jubilee World Tribute, 1949) found that not only were they well tolerated but children were happy to eat them. Over the following years, Dr Haas treated many cases of children with coeliac disease with his 'Specific Carbohydrate Diet', consisting not only of bananas but also of particular carbohydrate-containing fruit and vegetables. By keeping patients on the diet for a minimum of 12 months he found that the disease prognosis was excellent, with complete recovery, no relapse or mortality and normal growth. Haas was also the first to recognise the familial tendency to the disease, especially in identical twins (Haas, 1932).

In 1951, Dr Haas together with his son (Haas & Haas, 1951) published *The Management of Coeliac Disease*, the most comprehensive medical text yet written on coeliac disease and the first in which a specific carbohydrate diet was offered as an effective and lasting treatment, and moreover, one widely accepted as a cure for coeliac disease.

Protein versus carbohydrates

Whilst the Drs Haas were writing their book, a Dutch paediatrician Professor Dicke was completing his doctoral thesis (1950), in which he observed that removing wheat, oats and rye flour from the diet of children with coeliac disease dramatically improved their symptoms. His observation came as a result of the fluctuation in the supply of wheat flour in Holland after the Second World War.

Activity

If you have a coeliac patient who experienced the war years, ask them about their diet and health at that time.

What foods were rationed during and after the Second World War in Britain, and how were these substituted? Would the absence of some foodstuffs or their replacement with others have been likely to have had a positive or negative effect on those with coeliac disease?

As a consequence, rice or potato flour was used instead of wheat flour and Dicke observed that the clinical condition and faecal fat excretion of coeliac children on his ward varied considerably depending on the diet they were receiving. Further work with colleagues Professor Dolf Wijers and Jan Van de Kamer, not published until 1953 (Dicke *et al.*, 1953), identified the association between faecal fat excretion and changes in the ingredients of food between rice, potato and wheat and identified a factor in wheat as the main cause of the symptoms but acknowledged that this factor was not wheat starch. They surmised that the wheat factor thus far identified only in wheat, rye and oats probably existed in other foodstuffs not yet tested. In the meantime in 1952, a group of paediatricians and pharmacologists from Birmingham University had already published their report in *The Lancet* (Anderson *et al.*, 1952). Continuing on from Dicke's original (1950) extensive and intuitive work, they showed that indeed it was not the carbohydrate (starch) in grain that was the culprit in coeliac disease but the protein gluten in wheat and rye flour that caused the symptoms associated with the disease – this it appeared was the 'wheat factor'. Wheat flour and more specifically wheat gluten when reintroduced into the diet caused a deterioration in symptoms, whilst the reintroduction of wheat starch did not. Anderson (1952) and her colleagues concluded that the changes to gastrointestinal function in children with coeliac disease were very similar to those in adults with idiopathic steatorrhoea. However, the precise way in which the gluten fraction disturbed that function remained to be shown.

DEFINITION OF COELIAC DISEASE

From Cappadocia to Paris – children to adults

The link that Anderson (1952) and her colleagues made back to adult disease is important, as most of the key advances in our understanding of coeliac disease in the early twentieth century came from work with children, quite possibly because the children's response to the newly emerging treatments was the most dramatic. Although recognising that there were similarities, the disease in adults was deemed a distinct entity and thus termed adult coeliac disease, in addition to other terms such as coeliac sprue, idiopathic steatorrhoea and non-tropical sprue which were also reported. Although different terms were used to describe the disease in adults to that in children, the main source of confusion was not so much in the name as in the lack of clear defining criteria for diagnosing the disease.

Further studies of idiopathic steatorrhoea were undertaken by the Birmingham group (Cooke *et al.*, 1953) and the chronic nature of coeliac disease became increasingly appreciated. They proved that in almost a half of the cases of idiopathic steatorrhoea there was a definitive or presumptive history in infancy or childhood consistent with coeliac disease. Hence, the presentation and treatment of adult coeliac disease was acknowledged and the benefits of a gluten free diet became established in adults (French *et al.*, 1957).

As far back as 1910 studies into the histological appearances in the jejunum in idiopathic steatorrhoea had shown changes to the villi lining the small bowel, notably atrophy. Unfortunately, the fact that in these studies histology was obtained postmortem meant that the abnormalities were largely ignored as postmortem change (Paulley, 1954). As the links between these variously named diseases were established these histological findings would eventually form the basis of the diagnostic criteria that defined coeliac disease (see Table 1.1).

Table 1.1   Summary showing history of coeliac disease

Year	Contribution	By whom
Second century AD ⇓	The first known description of the disease with the predominant features of diarrhoea, pallor, weight loss and chronic relapse.	Aretaeus of Cappadocia
1856 ⇓	The translation of Aretaeus' work from Greek to Latin, printed for the Sydenham Society of London.	Francis Adams
1888 ⇓	The first recognition of its treatment being related to diet.	Dr Samuel Gee
1908 ⇓	The observation that whilst fats were tolerated moderately well, carbohydrates were poorly tolerated, almost always causing relapse or a return of diarrhoea.	Dr Emmett Holt and Christian Herter
1921 ⇓	The observation that carbohydrates particularly bread and cereals were the last foods that could be reintroduced into the diet and that growth suffered in proportion to the length of time that symptoms persisted.	Dr John Howland
1932 ⇓	The first recognition of a familial tendency to the disease especially in identical twins.	Dr Sydney Haas
Cited 1949 ⇓	The observation that children with severe diarrhoea did well on banana flour and plantain meal. The 'specific carbohydrate diet', consisting of bananas and particular carbohydrate containing fruit and vegetables, recognised as treatment.	Dr Sydney Haas
1950 ⇓	The observation that removing wheat, oats and rye flour from the diet of children with coeliac disease dramatically improved their symptoms.	Professor Dicke
1953 ⇓	Identified a factor in wheat as the main cause of the symptoms but acknowledged that this factor was not wheat starch.	Professor Dicke, Professor Dolf Wijers & Jan Van de Kamer
1952	Identified that the wheat factor was the protein gluten.	C. Anderson, J. French, H. Sammons, A. Frazer, J. Gerrard & J. Smellie

The first agreed definition

Coeliac disease continued to gain international acceptance. In 1968, The European Society for Paediatric Gastroenterology and Nutrition (ESPGAN) was founded following an inaugural meeting in Paris and an agreed definition of coeliac disease finally published in 1970 (Meuwisse, 1970). In order to make a definitive diagnosis there of course had to be a history and clinical presentation compatible with coeliac disease, ruling out other clinical conditions that might mimic the disease.

The diagnostic criteria required the fulfilment of three conditions:

1. A state of malabsorption with total or subtotal villous atrophy of the intestinal mucosa observed on a diet containing gluten.
2. A return to normal in the histological abnormalities and clinical condition on withdrawal of gluten from the diet.
3. A relapse in the histological abnormalities and clinical symptoms when once again challenged with a diet containing gluten.

This definition was rigorous in that it required small bowel biopsies on three separate occasions; nonetheless it enabled coeliac disease to be consistently and reliably diagnosed across countries and also across different research studies and therefore allowed the condition to be recognised as a distinct and separate entity from other, more transient, causes of small intestinal villous atrophy.

However, in clinical practice, reliance on the rather cumbersome, unreliable and patient-unfriendly Crosby capsule technique in obtaining these biopsies leads clinicians to question the need for the gluten challenge. Furthermore, when ESPGAN reviewed the criteria in 1978 (McNeish *et al.*, 1979), it became clear that unsurprisingly only two-thirds of its members were actually carrying out the gluten challenge seen as central to the definition of coeliac disease. It was suggested that the ESPGAN (Meuwisse, 1970) criteria were not required for the diagnosis of all patients, especially when they showed (McNeish *et al.*,

1979) that initial diagnosis was confirmed at the time of first biopsy in 95% of their patients. The criteria, however, at this time were not modified.

A revised definition

A further 10 years of experience in managing coeliac disease strengthened the call for a revision of the diagnostic criteria. New diagnostic tools, as will be described later, proved to be more reliable indicators of sensitisation to gluten and further larger studies using the ESPGAN criteria (Guandalini *et al.*, 1989) also suggested that in most cases the gluten challenge was unnecessary. ESPGAN recognised the progress in the diagnosis of coeliac disease since the publication of the initial definition and in 1990 published a 'simplified procedure' recommending that a gluten challenge was no longer mandatory (Walker-Smith *et al.*, 1990). The importance, however, of the initial diagnostic small bowel biopsy was emphasised and the subsequent clear-cut clinical improvement on a gluten free diet over weeks, not months, remained mandatory. Thus more fortunately for most coeliac patients a reliable diagnosis could now be made on the basis of one set of small bowel biopsies as opposed to three. However, it still recommended the biopsy capsule over the endoscope to ensure that a diagnostically adequate specimen was obtained.

The difficulty in the diagnosis of asymptomatic cases, such as first-degree relatives, was addressed by making a second biopsy on a gluten free diet essential in order to show mucosal recovery, as the absence of symptoms would otherwise make it impossible to monitor clinical improvement. A gluten challenge was still recommended in cases where a gluten free diet was commenced without an initial biopsy or where the initial biopsy did not show characteristic changes. Today, a gluten challenge is sometimes requested by patients who doubt their own diagnosis. This is especially seen with teenagers diagnosed with coeliac disease as children, embarking on a career pathway where their diagnosis is a barrier to entering certain professions.

Revising the definition further?

In completing this chapter looking at the history of the disease, an updated ESPGAN criterion for the diagnosis of coeliac disease has yet to be published. However, the simplified procedure described by Walker-Smith *et al.* (1990) is itself increasingly challenged from continued advances in the recognition of a spectrum of histological abnormalities as well as acceptance of a widening range of clinical presentations (some without gastrointestinal symptoms), the development of increasingly specific and sensitive antibody markers and the identification of genetic markers.

What the remainder of this book will show is that steatorrhoea is no longer the chief presenting symptom as described by Aretaeus or Gee. Certainly, over the years it has become apparent that 50–60% of individuals with this condition may be virtually asymptomatic or latent (Marsh, 1993) and even symptomatic individuals may present with atypical symptoms, such as neuropathy, arthropathy or simply vague ill health, all of which can and do frequently remain unrecognised. Any updated criterion for diagnosing coeliac disease in the future needs to take into account its many different aspects as a syndrome as apposed to a single entity.

HINTS AND TIPS

When developing information:

Consider developing a potted history of coeliac disease as information to give to patients at diagnosis. Not only is it good general interest but also it is a non-threatening opener to further information and education.

REFERENCES

Adams, F. (1856) *The Extant Works of Aretaeus the Cappadocian.* The Sydenham Society of England, London. www.chlt.

org/.../dh/aretaeusEnglish/index.html. Accessed 12 November 2006.

Anderson, C., French, J., Sammons, H., Frazer, A., Gerrard, J. & Smellie, J. (1952) Coeliac disease: Gastro-intestinal studies and the effect of dietary wheat flour. *The Lancet* 1(17):836–842.

Cooke, W.T., Peeney, A.L.P. & Hawkins, C.F. (1953) Symptoms, signs and diagnostic feature of idiopathic steatorrhea. *Quarterly Journal of Medicine* 22:59–77.

Dicke, W.K. (1950) Investigations of the harmful effects of certain types of cereal on patients with coeliac disease. Thesis, Utrecht.

Dicke, W.K., Weijers, H.A. & Van de Kamer, J.H. (1953) Coeliac disease: 11. The presence in wheat of a factor having a deleterious effect in cases of coeliac disease. *Acta Paediatrica* 42:34–42.

French, J.M., Hawkins, C.F. & Smith, N.M. (1957) The effect of wheat-gluten free diet in adults idiopathic steatorrhea. A study of 22 cases. *Quarterly Journal of Medicine* 26:481–499.

Gee, S. (1888) On the coeliac affliction. *St Bartholomew's Hospital Reports* 24:17–20.

Golden Jubilee World Tribute to Dr Sidney V Haas (1949) *The Story of Dr Sidney V Haas*. New York Academy of Medicine, New York.

Guandalini, S., Ventura, A., Ansadi, N., Giunta, A.M., Greco, L. & Lazzari, R. (1989) Diagnosis of coeliac disease: Time for a change? *Archives of Diseases in Childhood* 64:1320–1325.

Gull, W. (1855) Fatty stools from disease of the mesenteric glands. *Guy's Hospital Report* 1:369.

Haas, S.V. (1932) Coeliac disease: Its specific treatment and cure without nutritional relapse. *JAMA* 99(6):448–452.

Haas, S.V. & Haas, M.P. (1951) *Management of Coeliac Disease*. Lippincott Company, Philadelphia.

Herter, C.A. (1908) *On Infantilism from Chronic Intestinal Infection*. Macmillan, New York.

Marsh, M.N. (1993) Gluten sensitivity and latency: Can patterns of intestinal antibody secretion define the great 'silent majority?' (Editorials). *Gastroenterology* 104:1550–1553.

McNeish, A.S., Harms, K., Rey, J., Shmerling, D.H. & Walker-Smith, J.A. (1979) Re-evaluation of diagnostic criteria for coeliac disease. *Archives of Disease in Childhood* 54:783–786.

Meuwisse, G.W. (1970) Diagnostic criteria in coeliac disease. *Acta Paediatrica Scandinavica* 59:461.

Newland, J. (1921) Prolonged intolerance to carbohydrates. *Transactions of American Paediatric Society* 44:11.

Paulley, J.W. (1954) Observations of the aetiology of idiopathic steatorrhoea. *British Medical Journal* 4900:1318–1321.

Walker-Smith, J.A., Guandalini, S., Schmitz, J., Shmerling, D.H. & Visakorpi, J.K. (1990) Revised criteria for diagnosis of coeliac disease (report of the Working Group of European Society of Paediatric Gastroenterology and Nutrition). *Archives of Disease in Childhood* 65:909–911.

Chapter 2
The Characteristics of Coeliac Disease

LEARNING OUTCOMES

At the end of this chapter you should be able to:

- Describe the structure and function of the small bowel.
- Understand how it is that an immunological reaction can develop as a result of dietary exposure.
- Explain the triggers for and the nutritional significance of malabsorption in coeliac disease.
- Discuss the genetic links and their significance.

Coeliac disease is a complex immune-mediated syndrome primarily affecting the gastrointestinal tract with strong interactions between environmental and genetic factors. It is characterised by chronic inflammation, resulting in damage to the small intestinal mucosa, caused by the gliadin fraction of wheat gluten (glutamine) and similar proteins (prolamins) in barley and rye. The presence of gluten in the diet of those individuals with coeliac disease leads to self-perpetuating mucosal damage, whereas removal of gluten from the diet results in full mucosal recovery (Fasano & Cattasi, 2001).

With the prevalence of coeliac disease now thought to be between 1:100 and 1:200 in the UK population (Hourigan, 2006), it is increasing likely that nurses, whatever their area of practice or expertise, will at some point play a role in the care and management of these patients. Although complex, in order to understand how it is that an immunological reaction can develop as a result of dietary exposure, an understanding of the pathway leading to the production of antibodies to gliadin, tissue transglutaminase and endomysium is essential. It is also necessary to understand the normal structure and function of the small intestine to compare it with that characterising coeliac disease and its resultant malabsorption and it is here that we begin.

STRUCTURE AND FUNCTION OF THE SMALL INTESTINE

Structure

The small intestine (Figure 2.1) is a convoluted tube, approximately 6.5 m long. It occupies a large part of the abdominal

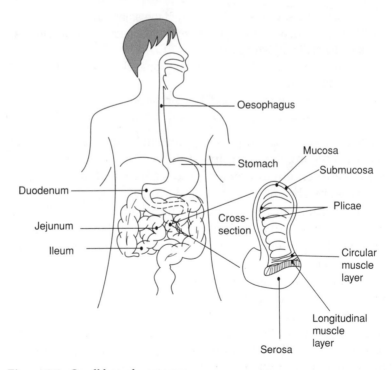

Figure 2.1 Small bowel anatomy.

cavity, starting at the pyloric sphincter and extending to the ileocaecal valve at the junction with the large intestine. It is suspended to the posterior abdominal wall by a fold of peritoneum called the mesentery, which allows free movement and rotation of the intestine and carries the nerves and the blood and lymphatic vessels that support the area.

The small intestine is the main area of digestion and absorption and is divided into three distinct anatomical areas:

1. The duodenum – At approximately 30 cm, this is the shortest segment of small intestine, extending from the pylorus to the jejunum at the ligament of Treitz. It forms a 'C'-shaped loop inferior to the stomach, enclosing the body of the pancreas. The duodenum itself is divided into two parts. The first part is called the bulb; the second part receives the bile and pancreatic juices from the ducts of the gall bladder and pancreas via the involuntary sphincter like muscle, the sphincter of Oddi. The duodenum plays a central role in controlling digestion.
2. The jejunum – At approximately 3.5 m, it extends from the duodenum to the ileum. As with the duodenum the main function of the jejunum is that of digestion.
3. The ileum – At approximately 2.5 m, it is the distal part of the small intestine connecting the small with the large intestine at the caecum via the ileocaecal valve, which prevents reflux of caecal contents. The ileum is the main area of absorption.

The blood supply to the small intestine is derived from the superior mesenteric artery, which supplies the intestine from the lower part of the duodenum. Venous drainage is via the superior mesenteric vein into the portal vein. Lymphatic drainage is into the thoracic duct via the mesenteric lymph nodes and ascending lymphoid channels.

The wall of the small intestine has the same composition as the remainder of the alimentary tract. Comprising a number of layers, described here from the outside inwards:

The serosa. Or adventitia, formed of peritoneum.
The muscular coat. This comprises a thin external layer of longitudinal fibres and a thicker internal layer of circular fibres.

Between these layers sits the myenteric (Auerbach's) plexus, which as part of the enteric nervous system provides motor innervation to both layers, i.e. allows movement and secretomotor innervation to the mucosa, i.e. induces gland secretion.

The submucosa. This contains blood vessels, lymph vessels and nerves. The duodenum contains compound tubular glands known as Brunner's glands, connected to the lumen by narrow ducts. The main function of these glands is to produce an alkaline mucous secretion that lubricates the intestinal walls and protects the intestine from the acidic content of chyme when it enters the duodenum from the stomach. By providing an alkaline condition for the intestinal enzymes to function this then enables absorption to take place. These glands are not found in the remainder of the small intestine.

The muscularis mucosae. A thin layer of smooth muscle separating the submucosa from the mucosa.

The mucosal layer. The mucosal layer comprises a layer of connective tissue known as the lamina propria and the epithelial lining. The lamina propria contains fibroblasts, macrophages, lymphocytes, neutrophils, mast cells and many other cells. The mucosal epithelium (Figure 2.1) is thrown into circular folds or plicae, which unlike the rugae of the stomach are permanent, increasing the area available for absorption. Projecting from these plicae are finger-like projections called villi. An arteriole, venule and a lymphatic channel known as a lacteal supply each villous. These villi then bear further projections called microvilli. At the base of the villi are intestinal glands known as the crypts of Lieberkuhn. These crypts are where the cell proliferation takes place and are also responsible for secreting various enzymes, including maltase and sucrase. In normal tissue the villi are at least twice as long as the depth of the crypts.

The epithelium of the small intestine also contains a number of distinct cell types:

Enterocytes. These make up most of the intestinal lining. These cells help break up molecules and transport them into the tissues. They are columnar, with a central nucleus. On the luminal surface, the microvilli are covered by glycoproteins, and attached mucins and enzymes, forming a prominent brush border, also known as the apical surface. There is a tight junction linking adjacent enterocytes which helps to separate the luminal surface of the intestine from the basal surface and stop pathogens from entering the basal surface.

Goblet cells. These are glandular simple columnar epithelial cells whose sole function is to produce and secrete mucin.

Paneth cells. These are found at the base of the crypts in the small intestine. They provide host defence against microbes in the small intestine by secreting antibacterial proteins when exposed to bacteria or bacterial antigens.

Enteroendocrine cells. Also known as neuroendocrine cells, these are found predominantly near the crypt bases and produce a number of different hormones mainly responsible for controlling gastrointestinal motility and secretion.

Stem cells. These are located just above the Paneth cell area. Stem cells are primal cells common to all multicellular organisms that retain the ability to renew themselves through cell division and differentiation, which is the acquisition of a cell type depending on the genetic activation. Here, they replenish the entire epithelium by dividing to produce one daughter stem cell and one daughter cell that proliferates, differentiates and migrates up the crypt.

The small intestine also contains considerable amounts of lymphoid tissue. Solitary lymphoid follicles or Peyer's patches are found throughout the mucous membrane but are found more prominently in the ileum. These follicles are observable to the naked eye as elongated thickenings of the intestinal epithelium measuring a few centimetres in length. They are situated in the mucosa, extending into the submucosa of the ileum. They are important in the immune surveillance of the lumen of the intestine and in facilitating the activation of the immune response within the mucosa.

Function

The small intestine is responsible for the chemical digestion and absorption of approximately 9 litres of fluid a day. On average, transit through all three sections of the small intestine takes 4–5 hours. During which time the small intestine will absorb approximately 7 litres of that fluid and the porridge-like consistency of the chyme entering the small intestine will be reduced to a thin watery mixture.

The small intestine is where most chemical digestion takes place. Peptides which are complex chains of protein molecules are broken down into amino acids; lipids (fats) are broken down into fatty acids and glycerol; and carbohydrates are broken down into simple sugars such as glucose. To achieve this chyme is mixed with digestive juices including bile, pancreatic juice and amylase and intestinal enzymes including maltase, lactase and sucrase; these break down the chyme and assist in the absorption of nutrients.

The villi and microvilli increase the overall absorptive surface area of the small intestine to around the area of a tennis court, providing extremely efficient absorption of nutrients. Inside each villous is a series of lacteals (lymph vessels) and capillaries. The lacteal lymph vessels absorb digestive fat into the lymphatic system which eventually drains into the bloodstream. The capillaries receive the other nutrients and transport them via the hepatic portal vein to the liver.

Coeliac disease is characterised by a flat mucosa with absent villi (villous atrophy) and elongated crypts (crypt hyperplasia) (Figure 2.2), compromising the absorptive surface area and leading to malabsorption. The significance of any nutrient deficiency is dependent on the absorptive area affected by the disease, which commences proximally in the duodenum and advances distally if the disease remains untreated.

Activity

Think about how you would explain to patients how destruction of the villi leads to malabsorption.

Malabsorption has a particularly detrimental effect on iron, fat and fat-soluble vitamin (A, D, E and K) uptake, and also affects the absorption of carbohydrates, certain salts and vitamin B. Their nutritional significance is outlined in Table 2.1.

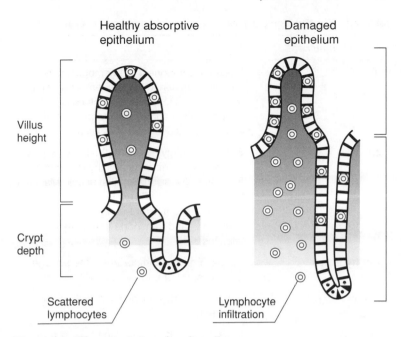

Figure 2.2 Characteristics of coeliac disease.

Nutrients that are mainly absorbed in the proximal small intestine such as iron and calcium are most affected by coeliac disease, whilst nutrients absorbed predominantly in the jejunum and ileum, such as folic acid, vitamin C and vitamin B12, are affected only when the disease is more advanced. There are of course other causes of malabsorption which should not be excluded (Figure 2.3).

How any of these nutritional deficiencies might impact on the symptoms of individuals with coeliac disease will become clearer when looking at disease presentation.

PATHOGENESIS OF COELIAC DISEASE

So, what are the key steps underlying the intestinal inflammatory response seen in coeliac disease? As already acknowledged, coeliac disease is a complex immune-mediated syndrome with strong interactions between environmental and genetic factors.

Table 2.1 The nutritional significance of malabsorption in coeliac disease

Macro/micro nutrient		*Significance*
Iron	$\Longrightarrow$	Essential component of haemoglobin as a carrier of oxygen to the tissues. As a transport medium for electrons within the cells (cytochromes) and as an integral part of enzyme reactions in various tissues.
Fats	$\Longrightarrow$	Serve as energy stores for the body. Play a vital role in maintaining healthy skin and hair. Insulate body organs against shock. Maintain body temperature. Promote healthy cell function. Essential for the digestion, absorption and transportation of fat-soluble vitamins.
Carbohydrates	$\Longrightarrow$	Simple molecules important in the storage and transport of energy.
Calcium	$\Longrightarrow$	A major mineral essential for healthy bones and teeth.
Vitamin A	$\Longrightarrow$	Essential for vision, developmental growth, cellular differentiation and proliferation, reproduction and in boosting the immune system.
Vitamin D	$\Longrightarrow$	Acts like a hormone, regulating the formation of bone and the absorption of calcium and phosphorus from the intestine. It helps to control the movement of calcium between bone and blood, and vice versa.
Vitamin E	$\Longrightarrow$	An antioxidant and is required by the body for many different functions including maintenance of cardiovascular health and the protection of cells, fatty acids and certain vitamins from oxidation. It also promotes normal blood clotting, the release of insulin from the pancreas, and skin regeneration.
Vitamin B	$\Longrightarrow$	As a group the B vitamins maintain healthy skin and muscle tone, enhance the function of the immune and nervous system and promote cell growth and division.
Vitamin K	$\Longrightarrow$	Necessary for the formation of prothrombin, required for blood clotting.

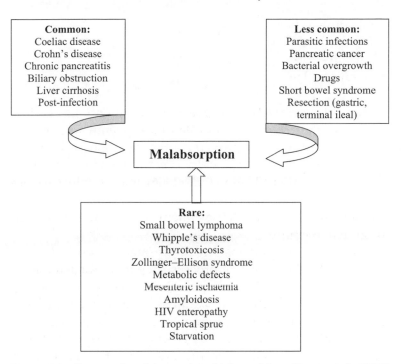

Common:	Less common:
Coeliac disease	Parasitic infections
Crohn's disease	Pancreatic cancer
Chronic pancreatitis	Bacterial overgrowth
Biliary obstruction	Drugs
Liver cirrhosis	Short bowel syndrome
Post-infection	Resection (gastric, terminal ileal)

Malabsorption

Rare:
Small bowel lymphoma
Whipple's disease
Thyrotoxicosis
Zollinger–Ellison syndrome
Metabolic defects
Mesenteric ischaemia
Amyloidosis
HIV enteropathy
Tropical sprue
Starvation

Figure 2.3 Causes of malabsorption. (Adapted from Travis *et al.*, 2005.)

The gliadin fraction of wheat gluten and similar proteins in other grains cause the immunological hypersensitivity to genetically susceptible individuals required for disease activation. Thanks to their discovery, as outlined in Chapter 1, these can now be used to turn off and on the immunological events responsible for the damage to the intestinal mucosa (Hollen, 2006).

Collectively, the disease-activating proteins in wheat, barley and rye are known as gluten. Strictly speaking, gluten is the cohesive mass that remains after washing wheat flour dough; however, gluten-like proteins are also found in rye, barley and, to a lesser extent, oats.

These proteins are either insoluble or soluble in alcohol, and it is the latter, known as prolamines, that are implicated in coeliac disease.

The disease-activating prolamines in the various cereals are:

- Gliadin – Wheat
- Hordein – Barley
- Secalin – Rye
- Avenin – Oats

The exclusion of oats has always been contentious possibly because of the lower level of prolamines. Avenin accounts for only 5–15% of the total protein content as opposed to a 40% gliadin content in wheat (Shewry *et al.*, 1992). However, there is some indication (Silano *et al.*, 2006) that certain varieties of oats may be potentially harmful to individuals with coeliac disease possibly because these patients have a lower threshold for gluten tolerance.

Prolamines are proteins which are made up of chains of amino acids. The digestive process prepares proteins for absorption by cutting these chains of amino acids into smaller chains known as peptides. Prolamines have high levels of proline and glutamine. The proline content renders these proteins resistant to degradation by gastric, pancreatic and brush border enzymes resulting in the presence of large peptides with a high proline and glutamine content in the small bowel (Hourigan, 2006; Kagnoff, 2005). These proline-rich fragments easily pass through the digestive system of normal individuals, but what happens in those with coeliac disease?

Genetics

It has been apparent for many years that there might be a heritable component to coeliac disease. Multiple cases of the disease have been identified within families, with first-degree relatives of patients with coeliac disease having a 10% greater prevalence than seen in the general population (AGA, 2006) and in monozygotic twins the concordance rate is about 80%.

There is a strong association to the major histocompatibility complex Class II (MHC Class II) antigen allele, HLA-DQ2. The majority of coeliac patients carry the gene that codes for this allele, and others carry the allele for HLA-DQ8. It is highly unlikely that just one gene is involved in determining disease susceptibility, particularly as these alleles can be found in 40% of the non-coeliac population (Hourigan, 2006). Further genetic studies are being done to determine other genes that could contribute to disease development.

Activity

Ask patients if there is a history of coeliac disease in their family? What might be the significance of this, thinking particularly about un-diagnosed disease? What might you advise?

What triggers the onset of coeliac disease?

How and when gluten sensitivity and the development of an autoimmune response first occur remains unknown. A variety of hypotheses have been forwarded including enteric infection or recent surgery resulting in a compromise of the epithelial barrier function (AGA, 2006). In addition, the early appearance of cereals into the infant diet may provoke an increased risk of developing childhood disease. It remains unknown to what extent delaying the introduction of gluten to infants 'at risk' of developing coeliac disease is beneficial (AGA, 2006). Minimising the delay in diagnosis remains important in terms of the health benefits to those individuals.

What happens when coeliac patients ingest gluten?

For those who enjoy the science, read on!

The interplay between genetics and the environmental factors of coeliac disease is not entirely understood. The following is based on what is currently known, although it is acknowledged that as our understanding grows some aspects of this 'cause and effect' story may change (Figure 2.4).

In genetically susceptible people the ingestion of gluten generates both an adaptive and an innate immune response.

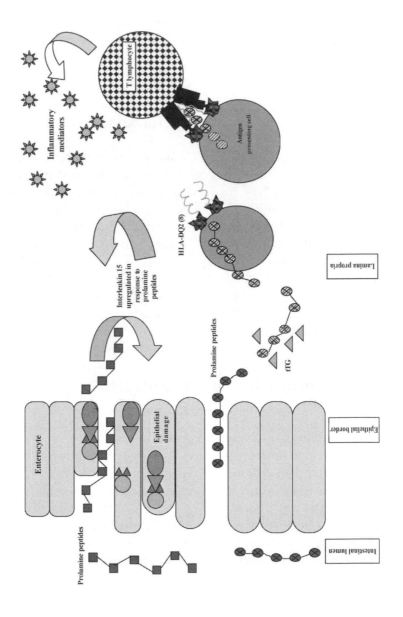

The adaptive immune response is triggered when prolamines (proline-rich, large, undigested peptides) within the small bowel cross the epithelial barrier to the lamina propria. Here, they are modified by a protein called tissue transglutaminase (tTG). tTG changes the glutamine within the prolamine to glutamic acid which makes prolamine particularly attractive to antigen-presenting cells (APCs) expressing the major histocompatibility complex HLA-DQ2. These highly specialised cells are able to 'digest' the peptide and then 'display' it (via the HLA-DQ2) to the lymphocytic T cells, CD4[+]. This action triggers an inflammatory response in the lamina propria possibly releasing mediators which cause tissue damage.

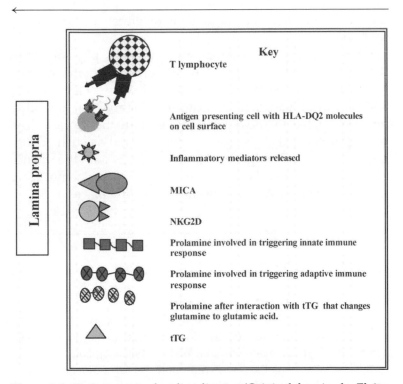

Figure 2.4 Pathogenesis of coeliac disease. (Original drawing by Elaine Horne.)

The presence of a prolamine peptide within the lumen of the small bowel will also cause activation of the innate immune system by the release of a cytokine, interleukin 15 (IL15). Studies suggest that this is in fact a different prolamine peptide than that which induces the activation of the adaptive immune response (involving APCs, HLA-DQ2 and T cells). Because of the enhanced expression of IL15, an MHC-type molecule named MICA is expressed on epithelial enterocytes together with the upregulation of a particular receptor (NKG2D) on intraepithelial lymphocytes (IELs). The interaction between the receptor (NKG2D) and MICA causes the destruction of the enterocytes leading to the characteristic blunting of the villi.

It is unlikely that the adaptive and innate immune responses proceed in isolation. It is entirely possible that inflammation in the lamina propria will upregulate IL15 and similarly the destruction of enterocytes and loss of epithelial integrity will make possible the movement of gluten to the lamina propria.

Understanding the normal anatomy and physiology of the small bowel is essential in understanding the mechanism behind the symptoms associated with coeliac disease and, in turn, translating this into information that is readily understandable to those individuals with the disease. The pathogenesis of the disease is emerging and as such changing with our knowledge, but getting to grips with the science is useful as we should never assume that patients do not want to know what caused their disease in the first place.

HINTS AND TIPS

When developing information:

Visual aids are invaluable for explaining to patients the pathogenesis behind coeliac disease and how that leads to malabsorption.

Source what materials are out there whilst building up your information/education compendium. Consider using some of the materials in this chapter to develop your own materials.

REFERENCES

American Gastroenterological Association (2006) AGA Institute Medical Position Statement on the diagnosis and management of coeliac disease. *Gastroenterology* 131:1977–1980.

Fasano, A. & Catassi, C. (2001) Current approaches to diagnosis and treatment of coeliac disease: An evolving spectrum. *Gastroenterology* 120:636–651.

Hollen, E. (2006) *Coeliac Disease in Childhood: On the Intestinal Mucosa and the Use of Oats*. Linkoping University, Faculty of Health Sciences, Unpublished dissertation No. 965.

Hourigan, C.S. (2006) The molecular basis of coeliac disease. *Clinical and Experimental Medicine* 6:53–59.

Kagnoff, M.F. (2005) Overview and pathogenesis of coeliac disease. *Gastroenterology* 128:510–518.

Shewry, P.R., Tatham, A.S. & Kasarda, D.D. (1992) Cereal protein and coeliac disease. In Marsh, M.N. (ed), *Coeliac Disease*. Blackwell Scientific Publication, Oxford, pp. 305–348.

Silano, M., Dessi, M., DeVincenzi, M. & Cornell, H. (2006) In vitro tests indicate that certain varieties of oats may be harmful to patients with coeliac disease. *Journal of Gastroenterology and Hepatology* 22:528–531.

Travis, S.P.L., Ahmad, T., Collier, J. & Steinhart, A.H. (2005) Small intestine. In *Pocket Consultant Gastroenterology*. Blackwell Publishing Ltd, Oxford, pp. 207–242.

Chapter 3
Presentation of Coeliac Disease

LEARNING OUTCOMES

At the end of this chapter you should be able to:

- Discuss the changes in disease presentation over time.
- Describe the more unusual disease presentations.
- Discuss the implications of screening an unsuspecting population for coeliac disease.
- Describe the nursing support this group of patients require at this time and how this is best delivered.

For many years, coeliac disease has been associated with weight loss, diarrhoea and malabsorption of nutrients. The classic picture is that originally described as paediatric syndrome, the wasted, pale, pot-bellied child, but for every so-called classic presentation there are many more patients with few or no symptoms.

Since coeliac disease was first described the clinical manifestations appear to be changing and it is becoming apparent that a host of disorders in many systems are aetiologically related to the presence of coeliac disease. Despite the improved tests and their increased availability, diagnosis remains difficult in some cases and likely only if we adopt a lower threshold for suspecting that coeliac disease may underlie many different clinical syndromes (Duggan, 2004).

This chapter looks at a conceptual model for coeliac disease and the changes in disease presentation, including some

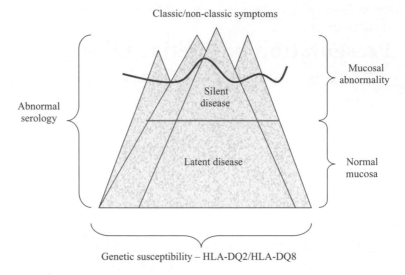

Figure 3.1   The coeliac iceberg.

more novel cases. The implications of recognising undetected coeliac disease at a general population level are uncertain but, as will become clear from the case study reported in this chapter, for some earlier diagnosis would certainly have made an appreciable difference to their quality of life.

CLASSIC AND NON-CLASSIC PRESENTATION

The coeliac iceberg

The coeliac iceberg is a model used to conceptualise how coeliac disease varies with respect to its clinical presentation and severity of symptoms. First introduced by Richard Logan in 1991 (Figure 3.1) and often referred to in the medical literature.

The base determines the overall size of the iceberg and the prevalence of coeliac disease, primarily influenced by those with the genetic susceptibility, DQ2 and/or DQ8. At the base are those healthy individuals who include gluten as part of their diet and have normal small bowel morphology even though they may have the same genetic constitution as those with coeliac disease.

The next layer of the iceberg describes those people with latent or preclinical disease – For example those who have a positive serological test but normal mucosa on a normal diet, but later may go on to develop symptoms or histological changes. Those with active disease also revert to this state when on a strict gluten free diet.

Next comes silent disease, incorporating those who have coeliac disease and yet display no overt symptoms. They are normally diagnosed as a result of screening, i.e. for family history or diabetes, or may present insidiously with mild degrees of iron deficiency anaemia, osteopenia or neurological symptoms.

The tip of the iceberg depicts the small proportion of the coeliac population with the typical 'classic' symptoms of the disease, diarrhoea, steatorrhoca, weight loss and failure to thrive. Those with clinical and silent disease have a typical small bowel lesion.

The waterline between the visible and submerged parts of the iceberg represents the ratio of diagnosed to undiagnosed cases, depending on such factors as awareness of the disease, availability of diagnostic facilities and exposure to gluten. Because the relevance of these factors varies according to population demographics, the waterline is much more unstable than the overall size of the iceberg, which explains the wide fluctuations reported in the incidence of the disease over the years (Fasano & Catassi, 2001).

Activity

Look at the presenting history of a coeliac patient, bearing in mind their symptoms and results of serological testing. Where on the iceberg would you place them?

The tip of the iceberg

The onset of the so-called 'classic' symptoms was always thought to occur most commonly in children between the ages of 6 and 24 months. Characterised by chronic diarrhoea, anorexia, failure to thrive, abdominal distension and muscle wasting, the stools being characteristically pale, loose, bulky and highly offensive (steatorrhoea) as a result of fat malabsorption. Although now rarer, in some cases the diarrhoea is so profuse that it leads to dehydration, hypokalaemia and acidosis, the so-called coeliac crisis, reported historically (Gee, 1888) as ultimately leading to death.

Now adult presentations are more common than paediatric presentations, the most common age being between 40 and 50 years (Mendoza, 2005). This is possibly in response to changing environmental stimuli such as encouraging mothers to breast-feed for longer and to wean infants on gluten free foods. The classic symptoms of coeliac disease are described in the adult population as affecting those mainly in their thirties and forties (Van Heel & West, 2006), characterised by diarrhoea, steatorrhoea and weight loss. But in contrast to childhood coeliac disease, adult disease usually has a more insidious onset with a wider spectrum of clinical manifestations. The commonest feature in more than two-thirds of adult patients is iron deficiency anaemia, with iron deficiency being the only abnormality in 40% of this group (Unsworth *et al.*, 1999), making it in theory the new 'classic' presentation, or in fashion terms the new black.

Activity

Find out what the normal investigative pathway for iron deficiency anaemia is within your clinical area or speciality. Does it include serological testing for coeliac disease?

However, there are case reports of adults presenting in coeliac crisis (Ozaslan *et al.*, 2004; Sanders *et al.*, 2005), showing that coeliac disease should not be ignored as a differential diagnosis in adults presenting with severe acute diarrhoea in combination with other symptoms such as weight loss and acidosis.

Above or below the waterline?

So with the considerable advances in our understanding of coeliac disease has come the recognition that those with adult disease do not always complain of the classic gastrointestinal symptoms, with a prevalence in classic malabsorptive presentation ranging from 1:2000 to 1:10 000 in the West (Schuppan & Junker, 2007), but neither do they all present with symptoms of iron deficiency. Increasingly, studies are showing a changing presentation with the diagnosis of coeliac disease being made on individuals with silent or atypical symptoms (Rampertab *et al.*, 2006; Winson *et al.*, 2003) and it is the difference between them being diagnosed or not that places them above or below the waterline of the coeliac iceberg.

The increase in the number of people with coeliac disease is not that more people are developing the disease but that improved and more accurate serological markers and our knowledge of the genetic links and increased access to endoscopic examinations are leading to more individuals being screened, investigated and as a result diagnosed (Sanders *et al.*, 2002; Van Heel & West, 2006), but it is estimated that it remains undiagnosed in 1% of the population (Van Heel & West, 2006).

Atypical presentations

Given that clinicians still fail to consider coeliac disease even when individuals present with classic symptoms (Rampertab *et al.*, 2006), the challenge remains in recognising the 'silent' majority. Nevertheless, the atypical presentations of coeliac disease reported in the medical press all help to raise awareness and lower the threshold of suspicion. Here a few such papers are highlighted.

Certainly few clinicians would expect obesity to be part of the presentation. Yet Furse and Mee (2005) describe four such cases as a reminder that as almost a quarter of men and women in the United Kingdom are now clinically obese with a body mass index (BMI) > 30, coeliac disease should not be excluded on the basis of weight. All the cases reported are female with BMIs of between 38 and 42. Two of the four were found to have iron deficiency anaemia and two also had a history of diarrhoea and irregular bowel habit, one of whose father had recently been diagnosed with the disease. All of these have already been discussed as the classic, new-classic or familial links, and identified by taking a careful history, but one of the four cases was that of a woman with a longstanding history of indigestion-type symptoms. A careful history in this case highlighted that her symptoms were worse with alcohol and bread. We could assume that at least in part her weight would be contributing to her symptoms, but interestingly on a gluten free diet her weight remained unchanged but her symptoms resolved entirely. Although historically associated with weight loss, we know that malabsorption of nutrients is dependent on the area of small bowel damage which tends to be greater proximally extending distally when the disease remains unchecked; therefore, these patients were probably able to use still intact absorptive mechanisms distally.

The complications associated with coeliac disease usually occur after many years of exposure to gluten and therefore the disease may remain silent until the complications manifest themselves, which is of course undesirable. Bennett *et al.* (2004) describe two cases both presenting with deteriorating night vision, with histories of looking through a coloured screen. Both on careful history also complained of diarrhoea/steatorrhoea and weight loss. Both were found to have vitamin deficiencies, and in particular vitamin A of which the basic molecule is retinol, a fat-soluble vitamin that cannot be absorbed through damaged intestinal mucosa. Night blindness is often the earliest manifestation of vitamin A deficiency and is reversible; the late changes cause permanent corneal damage and visual loss. Both patients were found to have coeliac disease and in both cases the night blindness improved rapidly on a gluten free diet and parental vitamins.

Another novel presentation described is that of three women who sought medical advice because of symptoms noted after stopping the Atkins diet (Van Heel & West, 2006). The Atkins diet recommends unlimited protein and fat intake with an initially restricted carbohydrate intake; the maintenance diet remains low in the cereal grains wheat, barley and rye – those toxic in coeliac disease. Two of the women were already known to have treated autoimmune hypothyroidism: one with an additional hypoadrenalism, and the third had no known concomitant disease. All three commenced the Atkins diet with its low carbohydrate intake, noticing increased well-being on this regimen. All then noticed increasing ill health with symptoms including tiredness, abdominal distension, pain and flatulence when they reintroduced bread into their diet. All were subsequently found to have coeliac disease and all three responded well to the gluten free diet.

Symptoms induced by gluten ingestion are often more marked after a period following a gluten free diet than the symptoms experienced prior to diagnosis and treatment (Van Heel & West, 2006). As the authors concluded any occurrence of gastrointestinal symptoms after following an Atkins-type low-carbohydrate diet should prompt investigation for coeliac disease.

Activity

What are the principles of the Atkins diet? In what way does it change the body's metabolism?

CLINICAL DISORDERS ASSOCIATED WITH COELIAC DISEASE

There are a myriad of clinical disorders associated with coeliac disease (Box 3.1).

The fact that it remains underdiagnosed is in part because it is not considered in those people at high risk or in clinical conditions that may be manifestations of coeliac disease (Murray, 2005). Several of the conditions mentioned (Box 3.1) have been described as having an association with coeliac disease that may be greater than by chance alone with certain autoimmune conditions such as insulin-dependent diabetes mellitus (type 1), hypothyroidism or dermatitis herpetiformis carrying an increased risk of coexisting coeliac disease (Murray, 2005). There is also evidence (Ventura *et al.*, 1999) to suggest that the prevalence of autoimmune diseases amongst those with coeliac disease is proportional to the time exposed to gluten before being diagnosed.

This section describes a selection of the conditions where there is evidence of an association with coeliac disease. By no

Box 3.1 Clinical disorders associated with coeliac disease (taken from Duggan, 2004)

1. Liver disease
2. Recurrent aphthous mouth ulcers
3. Lymphocytic gastritis
4. Reflux oesophagitis
5. Adenocarcinoma of the small bowel
6. Peripheral neuropathy
7. Epilepsy
8. Ataxia
9. Myelopathy
10. Depression
11. Schizophrenia
12. Type 1 diabetes
13. Infertility in men and women
14. Recurrent abortion
15. Thyroid disorders
16. Addison's disease
17. IgA deficiency
18. Anaemia (iron, folate and B12 deficiency)
19. Coagulation disorders (associated with vitamin K deficiency)
20. Hyposplenism
21. T-cell lymphoma
22. Osteopenia/osteoporosis
23. Arthralgia/arthritis
24. Dermatitis herpetiformis
25. Psoriasis
26. Dental defects
27. Down's syndrome
28. Cardiomyopathy

means exhaustive, it highlights some of the conditions where nurses might look more closely at the possibility of coeliac as a concomitant disorder, especially where there are ongoing symptoms or apparent treatment failures.

- Dermatitis herpetiformis
- Type 1 diabetes
- Osteoporosis
- Iron deficiency anaemia
- Infertility
- Neurological disease
- Hepatobiliary disorders

Activity

The next time you come across a patient with one of the following conditions where there is a possibility of treatment failure, look at whether coeliac disease has been considered as a concomitant disorder.

Dermatitis herpetiformis

Dermatitis herpetiformis is a lifelong, gluten-sensitive, blistering skin disease (Case study 3.1) first described and named by Dr Louis Duhring, an American dermatologist, in 1884 (Zone, 2005). It was J.B. van der Meer in Holland who first described the granular IgA deposited in dermal papillary tips (Van der Meer, 1969), now recognised as the hallmark of the disorder and a requirement for a definitive diagnosis. All patients with dermatitis herpetiformis have some degree of coeliac disease and are likely to reflect the entire spectrum seen in histological and clinical coeliac disease in adults, including the complications and course of the disease (Zone, 2005). The prevalence of HLA-DQ2 and DQ8 is also the same in coeliac disease as is the familial tendency (Zone, 2005).

Characteristic involvement is of pruritic papulovesicles and excoriations on the scalp, elbows, knees and buttocks. Patients with dermatitis herpetiformis will rarely have the classic symptoms of malabsorption but they all have the villous atrophy or at least inflammatory changes in the small bowel mucosa (gluten enteropathy), and both these changes and the cutaneous disease appear to respond well to a gluten free diet (Garioch *et al.*, 1994). The majority will have silent coeliac disease. Unlike patients with coeliac disease, those with dermatitis herpetiformis have an alternative treatment option. The cutaneous disease clears rapidly on treatment with Dapsone, a sulphone antibiotic medication, but recurs rapidly if the drug is discontinued. This has meant that some patients have chosen to take Dapsone long term and not restrict their gluten intake, despite knowing that gluten is the cause of their cutaneous disease. Whilst we do not know the long-term impact of such a strategy, Dapsone is not without its side effects, including potentially serious blood disorders on long-term treatment, and patients should be advised accordingly to allow them to make an informed decision.

Type 1 diabetes

It was over 40 years ago that the association between childhood diabetes mellitus and coeliac disease was recognised (Walker-Smith & Grigor, 1969), following on from which several studies in both children and adults showed a prevalence of coeliac disease of up to almost 7% in type 1 diabetes (Holmes, 2000). This association is probably due to both diseases having the common genetic predisposition HLA-DQB1, present in the majority of patients with both conditions. There is evidence that undiagnosed coeliac disease not only coexists with diabetes but may precede it and that delaying the diagnosis of coeliac disease may increase the risk for subsequently developing type 1 diabetes mellitus (Murray, 2005). Autoantibodies directed against islet cells are frequently present in untreated coeliac disease but disappear with a gluten free diet (Ventura *et al.*, 2000).

In about 90% of cases, diabetes is diagnosed first, probably because type 1 diabetes mellitus generally has an acute onset, which is easily identifiable from early symptoms. The varied and atypical presentation of coeliac disease is very often missed or symptoms of ill health are attributed to the already diagnosed diabetes. It is suggested (Holmes, 2000) that given the high prevalence and potentially correctable health risks of coeliac disease, screening of all patients with type 1 diabetes mellitus for coeliac disease would be preferable to a case-by-case approach, which would miss those with silent or atypical symptoms. However, patients already having to contend with a diabetic diet would also have to contend with a second, gluten free, diet and this needs careful monitoring by a registered dietitian. So, whatever position is adopted it is imperative that patients are given appropriate education and support to deal with a dual diagnosis that will have a profound effect on their dietary requirements.

Unexplained osteoporosis

Skeletal health is maintained by a continuous process of bone removal (resorption) and bone replacement (formation). An imbalance between the two can lead to osteoporosis or reduced bone mineral density (BMD). Low bone density is frequently seen in newly diagnosed patients with coeliac disease, especially in those presenting over the age of 40 years. Bone mass increases with age reaching its maximum between the ages of 25 and 30 years, after which time calcium intake and physical activity become vital in maintaining skeletal health. As we know, the most common age for the diagnosis of coeliac disease is 40–50 years (Mendoza, 2005), when bone mass has passed its peak. It also coincides with the age of menopause in women and an increased rate of bone resorption and decreased rate of bone replacement.

People with undiagnosed or untreated coeliac disease will generally have a reduced ability to absorb both calcium and vitamin D. They may also have a lactose intolerance hindering the absorption of calcium (Murray, 2005). Coupled with an increased bone turnover, this can lead to a lower BMD and osteoporosis.

Low bone density associated with coeliac disease responds to a gluten free diet, gradually improving BMD (Walters & Van Heel, 2003); however, a normal range is not always attained (Meyer *et al.*, 2001). In addition to the delayed diagnosis into adult life, this may, in part, be due to the fact that the gluten free diet itself has the potential to reduce an individual's calcium intake, with a tendency to eat less bread and also drink less milk because of the reduction in breakfast cereal eaten. Bread and cereals contribute for as much as 25% of the dietary calcium (Gregory *et al.*, 1990).

In the same way as coeliac disease, osteoporosis can run a silent course presenting only with bone fractures. Osteoporosis is now thought to be the most important long-term medical concern for those with coeliac disease (Walters, 2007) and so screening newly diagnosed coeliac patients for signs of reduced BMD is vital to provide a baseline for education, treatment and support. However, screening for coeliac disease in all patients with reduced BMD has been shown to have a low yield in the absence of gastrointestinal symptoms or anaemia (Sanders *et al.*, 2005) but should certainly be considered in older adults with unexplained metabolic bone disease.

> ### Activity
>
> Find out what the criteria are within your trust for screening patients for osteoporosis.

Iron deficiency anaemia

Iron is absorbed by the proximal small intestine, the site, as already described, of the greatest damage in coeliac disease. Therefore, it is perhaps unsurprising that iron deficiency anaemia is the commonest presenting feature in coeliac disease, occurring in over two-thirds of adult patients and as the only abnormality in 40% of this group (Unsworth *et al.*, 1999). This group of patients will be unresponsive to oral iron medication due to malabsorption. Iron deficiency is common in the general population but it is still surprising to note a number of older adults presenting with coeliac disease whom it transpires have been iron deficient for many years. In the case of females, it was often attributed to excessive menstrual loss or, if complaining of excessive tiredness, to the 'stress' of raising a family.

What is not clearly understood is why not all those with coeliac disease are iron deficient. As with other nutrients the variation in the extent of involvement of the small intestine may lead to some compensation in absorption, already discussed in relation to coeliac disease presenting in obese individuals. There is also an association between the genes that cause haemochromatosis (a genetic disorder resulting in iron overload) and coeliac disease. With the haemochromatosis-associated gene C282Y found to be more common in individuals with coeliac disease, resulting in higher haemoglobin and iron stores (Butterworth *et al.*, 2002).

From the author's own 5-year experience of running an iron deficiency anaemia service, it became obvious that historically endoscopists were not obtaining duodenal biopsies in those patients undergoing endoscopic investigation for anaemia, an observation made by others (Murray, 2005), thus potentially leading to delays in diagnosis and often multiple endoscopic procedures. As with the other conditions already described coeliac disease should be considered in patients with unexplained iron deficiency anaemia and duodenal biopsies should always be obtained on any patient undergoing endoscopic investigation for anaemia.

Infertility

Infertility may also be the first clinical manifestation of coeliac disease. It was first noted in the 1970s that when women with fertility problems were found to have coeliac disease that the problems resolved on a gluten free diet (Morris *et al.*, 1970).

More recently, studies (Collin *et al.*, 1996; Meloni *et al.*, 1999) have shown that the prevalence of undiagnosed coeliac disease in women attending infertility clinics is in the range of 3–4%, a significantly higher prevalence than that found in the general population, noted to be around 1.06%. Once pregnant, associations between untreated coeliac disease and a higher incidence of termination, miscarriage, babies with low birth weight or intrauterine growth retardation have also raised concern (Goddard & Gillett, 2006). Maternal coeliac disease diagnosed before birth was not associated with adverse fetal outcomes (Van Heel & West, 2006).

Given the increasing trend of having children later in life, this may prove to be a significant issue for many women and shows that coeliac disease should be considered as a cause of unexplained infertility, and as will be discussed later once diagnosed mean that these women will need additional education and support throughout the pregnancy.

Neurological disease

Coeliac disease has been associated with a number of neurological and psychiatric conditions including epilepsy, neuropathy, cerebellar ataxia, depression, tension and headache/migraine. Whereas the association was thought to be as a complication of coeliac disease, it is now increasingly recognised as an initial manifestation of the disease (Bushara, 2005). It has been suggested that neurological disease associated with gluten sensitivity results from the malabsorption of vitamins such as E, B6, B12 and folic acid, all known to play an important role in maintaining neurological health (Pengiran *et al.*, 2002). However, with some individuals presenting without gastrointestinal symptoms and with no mucosal abnormality on biopsy, it is thought by some to be more likely that these neurological disorders result from an immune response aimed at neural tissue antigens triggered by the ingestion of gluten (Hadjivassiliou *et al.*, 1999). Hadjivassiliou and colleagues (1999) observed an increase in antibodies directed against cerebellar tissue (anti-Purkinje cell antibodies) in patients presenting with cerebellar disease, which disappeared in most within 6 months of commencing a gluten free diet. Purkinje cells are some of the largest neurons in the human brain. There is moreover a link between the duration of neurological symptoms and the diagnosis of coeliac disease. Where there is evidence of progressive peripheral nerve and central nervous system damage, a gluten free diet will only show symptomatic improvement over a long time span and in some cases will achieve only a stabilisation of symptoms, for example less reliance on medication and fewer seizures in cases of epilepsy rather than a complete resolution. In these patients, it is suggested (Hadjivassiliou *et al.*, 1999) that there is probably marked Purkinje cell loss, cells which do not regenerate.

This remains a controversial area (Bushara, 2005), with questions as to whether gluten sensitivity contributes to the pathogenesis of neurological disease or whether it represents an epiphenomenon. If, however, there is a risk that a delayed diagnosis results in permanent neurological impairment then it is prudent to undertake serological tests to exclude coeliac disease in patients with unexplained neurological dysfunction.

Hepatobiliary disorders

It was almost 30 years ago that liver changes were first recognised in coeliac disease (Hagander *et al.*, 1977). In some cases, the changes seen in liver function are reversed on commencing a gluten free diet, whilst in others, where the liver disease is clinically significant, it is not amenable to dietary treatment. As with many of the other disorders discussed, it is unclear as to whether it is a complication, or a clinical manifestation, of coeliac disease, and both are described. Freeman (2006) reports cases where almost 10% of individuals with unexplained elevations of liver enzymes were found to have coeliac disease. He also reports (Freeman, 2006) cases where up to 60% of patients with known coeliac disease were found to have abnormal liver enzymes.

Abnormal liver enzymes may reflect a common immunopathogenesis with coeliac disease, as has been discussed with other diseases such as diabetes and hypothyroidism. Examples of immune-mediated liver disease include primary biliary cirrhosis, sclerosing cholangitis and autoimmune hepatitis. In most cases, an exact genetic predisposition has yet to be identified (Freeman, 2006).

In some, a common genetically based disorder may be responsible. For example, in haemochromatosis which leads to the inappropriate absorption of iron from the proximal small intestine (the site most commonly affected histologically by coeliac disease), a case is reported (Heneghan *et al.*, 2000) where treatment of an individual with coeliac disease resulted in worsening liver function, with eventual recognition of haemochromatosis as the cause, probably as a result of pathological improvement in the proximal small intestine and increased iron uptake (Freeman, 2006).

Chronic changes in liver enzymes may also result as a direct impact of coeliac disease. In cases where impaired absorption leads to malnutrition, this may also result in the deposition of fat in the liver (hepatic steatosis), related partly to reduced fat mobilisation from the hepatocytes (Freeman, 2006).

To screen or not to screen?

So with the increasing recognition that coeliac disease is more common than previously suspected, as highlighted in this section, questions arise about the value of population screening. Coeliac disease meets all of the five criteria put forward by the

World Health Organization (Wilson & Junger, 1968) in relation to the prerequisites for an effective screening programme.

1. There should exist individuals at increased risk from the disease – this we know to be approximately 1:300.
2. There should be convincing evidence that screening is effective in reducing cancer morbidity and mortality – treatment is effective in reducing the risk of long-term complications including lymphoma and other cancers.
3. The screening procedure should be practical and feasible – serological tests and endoscopy are readily available.
4. The cost of screening should be reasonable – tests especially serological tests are cost-effective.
5. The yield of screening tests must result in earlier diagnosis of the disease with a subsequent better survival of the identified patients – we know that increasingly the diagnosis of coeliac disease is being made on individuals presenting with long-term complications.

Although it appears to tick all of the boxes required for an effective screening programme, what is not addressed is the effects on the quality of life of asymptomatic individuals. Quality of life has to take into consideration the social and psychological aspects of well-being in addition to the physical. In other words what cannot be ignored, as espoused by Bowling (1997), is:

> . . . how the patient feels, rather than how doctors think they ought to feel on the basis of clinical measurements. . . .and, particularly where people are treated for chronic or life threatening conditions, the therapy has to be evaluated in terms of whether it is more or less likely to lead to an outcome of life worth living in social and psychological, as well as physical terms (p. 1).

Activity

How do the principles of screening for coeliac disease compare and differ from those undergoing screening for cancers (breast, cervical, bowel)? Think about the provision of information and support and how this group of patients might frame their health in comparison to those undergoing screening for cancer.

What is becoming evident (Collin, 2005) is that the health improvements experienced by screen-detected coeliac patients in the first year of diagnosis may not continue in the longer term, with many patients failing to continue to comply with a gluten free diet (Bardella *et al.*, 1994). The reasons will be discussed later, but obviously underline the necessity of the long-term follow-up of this patient group. It also questions the quality of life experienced by asymptomatic patients as a result of this diagnosis, when the natural history of symptom-free or screen-detected coeliac disease remains poorly understood.

The question is perhaps not one of the importances of mass screening but of the early recognition of those most at risk of coeliac disease. Nurses, in whatever clinical setting, are often best placed to recognise these patients and highlight the need for screening of those where the index of suspicion is highest.

The case study reported in this chapter highlights one such protracted disease course and underlines the need for clinical vigilance.

HINTS AND TIPS

When identifying your potential specialist population and education needs:

- Look at patients with known coeliac disease in your speciality, what do the patterns of referral look like? Can you see any areas that are particularly weak in identifying susceptible individuals and would benefit from additional information and/or education, i.e. an informal talk to a group of midwives in the authors trust proved invaluable in highlighting presentation in pregnancy and improved interdisciplinary working with existing patients during pregnancy?
- What is the position on local population screening in your area? Is this group of patients sufficiently supported through the process bearing in mind the potential impact? If not, what can be done to improve this?

Case study

A 79-year-old lady Mrs B moved to be nearer to her youngest daughter. Having registered with her local GP practice, routine blood tests revealed an iron deficiency anaemia. On questioning, she calmly stated that she had been anaemic almost throughout her adult life. It would appear that over numerous years she had attended her then GP complaining of feeling constantly tired. There was no weight loss although her weight was always low at around eight stone and she denied any bowel problems and as a consequence it had been put down to raising eight children which she had given birth to over a 12-year time span and running a home! Her visits over the years were normally to get a 'tonic' of some sort to help her cope with what had by then been termed as chronic fatigue.

Her husband had been a coach driver, frequently spending time away from home. According to Mrs B, he often became frustrated on his return home to find his wife unable to keep the house tidy; at times she became so tired that she simply did not have any energy to do anything. As the years progressed and the children became older, the relationship with her husband became more difficult. He started spending less time away from home and as a consequence became less tolerant of what he considered her increasing laziness. Eventually she discovered that he was having an affair and they divorced. Mrs B always considered this to be her own fault and responsibility and struggled on. In her sixties she started to notice tremors particularly in her hand and then suddenly her speech became slurred. Her GP suspected that she might have had a CVA and arranged an MRI scan which was normal. Her symptoms seemed at the time to improve and so she declined any further tests, still maintaining a guilt complex that she was somehow responsible for the burden that she had been and was becoming on her family; she became increasingly reclusive and her children became concerned at her health and apparent depression. Eventually, her younger daughter persuaded her to move closer to her.

The GP having discovered an iron deficiency picture persuaded her to undergo investigations despite the longstanding nature of her problems. Although reluctant she agreed to attending an outpatient appointment at the iron deficiency anaemia clinic and following a thorough history, examination and bloods agreed to having an upper GI endoscopy. At the time she refused bowel investigations. Bloods revealed a positive EMA titre and this was explained to Mrs B as indicating a possible cause for her symptoms. She underwent her upper GI endoscopy with duodenal biopsies, which revealed a MARSH 3 coeliac disease with subtotal villous atrophy. Mrs B was understandably anxious when the diagnosis was discussed with her and her daughter; careful explanation and ongoing dietetic support was ensured whilst she came to grips with the gluten free diet. Within 3 months Mrs B reported feeling like a new woman at the age of 80! Her mood had lifted, her tremors were far less marked and her energy levels had increased. Although she was struggling to cope with the diet when eating out, she was very excited at the new lease of life and determined to get everything right. DEXA scan unsurprisingly revealed osteoporosis but SBFT was normal. At her last appointment she said that she did wonder whether things might have been different had she been diagnosed all those years earlier and indeed whether she might still be married.

REFERENCES

Bardella, M.T., Molteni, N., Prampolini, L., Glunta, A.M., Baldassarri, A.R., Morganti, D. & Bianchi, P.A. (1994) Need for follow up in coeliac disease. *Archive of Diseases in Childhood* 70:211–213.

Bennett, D.H., Webster, G.J.M., Molyneux, P., Descamps, M.J.L., Plant, G.T. & Pereira, S.P. (2004) The world through tinted glasses. *The Lancet* 364(9431):388.

Bowling, A. (1997) The conceptualization of functioning, health and quality of life. In *Measuring Health. A Review of Quality of Life Measurement Scales*, 2nd edn. Open University Press, Maidenhead, pp. 1–8.

Bushara, K.O. (2005) Neurologic presentation of celiac disease. *Gastroenterology* 126:S92–S97.

Butterworth, J.R., Cooper, B.T., Rosenberg, W.M., Purkiss, M., Jobson, S., Hathaway, M., Briggs, D., Howell, W.M., Wood, G.M., Adams, D.H. & Iqbal, T.H. (2002) The role of haemochromatosis susceptibility gene mutations in protecting against iron deficiency anaemia in coeliac disease. *Gastroenterology* 123:444.

Collin, P. (2005) Should adults be screened for coeliac disease? What are the benefits and harms of screening? *Gastroenterology* 128:S104–S108.

Collin, P., Vilska, S., Heinonen, P.K., Hallstrom, O. & Pikkarainen, P. (1996) Infertility and coeliac disease. *Gut* 39:382–384.

Duggan, J. (2004) Coeliac disease: The great imitator. *Medical Journal of Australia* 180(10):524.

Fasano, A. & Catassi, C. (2001) Current approaches to diagnosis and treatment of celiac disease: An evolving spectrum. *Gastroenterology* 120:636–651.

Freeman, H.J. (2006) Hepatobiliary and pancreatic disorders in celiac disease (Editorial). *World Journal of Gastroenterology* 12(10):1503–1508.

Furse, R.M. & Mee, A.S. (2005) Atypical presentation of coeliac disease. *British Medical Journal* 330:773–774.

Garioch, J.J., Lewis, H.M. & Sargent, S.A. (1994) 25 years' experience of a gluten free diet in the treatment of dermatitis herpetiformis. *British Journal of Dermatology* 131:541–545.

Gee, S. (1888) On the coeliac affliction. *St Bartholomew's Hospital Reports* 24:17–20.

Goddard, C.J.R. & Gillett, H.R. (2006) Complications of coeliac disease, are all patients at risk? *Post Medical Journal* 92(973):705–712.

Gregory, J., Foster, K., Tyler, H. & Wiseman, M. (1990) *The Dietary and Nutritional Survey of British Adults*. Her Majesty's Stationery Office, London.

Hadjivassiliou, M., Chattopadhyay, A.K., Gibson, A., Lobo, A.J. & Smith, C.M.L. (1999) The role of gluten sensitivity in neurological illness. *CME Journal of Gastroenterology, Hepatology and Nutrition* 2(1):3–5.

Hagander, B., Berg, N.O., Brandt, L., Norden, A., Sjolund, K. & Stenstam, M. (1977) Hepatic injury in adult coeliac disease. *The Lancet* 2:270–272.

Heneghan, M.A., Feeley, K.M., Little, M.P. & McCarthy, C.F. (2000) Precipitation of iron overload and hereditary haemochromatosis after successful treatment of coeliac disease. *American Journal of Gastroenterology* 95:298–300.

Holmes, G.K.T. (2000) Coeliac disease and type 1 diabetes mellitus. *Diabetic Medicine* 18:169–177.

Logan, R.F. (1991) Problems and pitfalls in epidemiological studies of coeliac disease. *Dynamics Nutrition Research* 2:14–22.

Meloni, G.F., Dessole, S., Varigiu, N., Tomasi, P.A. & Musumeci, S. (1999) The prevalence of coeliac disease in infertility. *Human Reproduction* 14:2759–2761.

Mendoza, N. (2005) Coeliac disease: An overview of the diagnosis, treatment and management. *British Nutrition Foundation Bulletin* 30:231–236.

Meyer, D., Stavropolous, S. & Diamond, B. (2001) Osteoporosis in a North American adult population with coeliac disease. *American Journal of Gastroenterology* 96:112–119.

Morris, J.S., Adjukiewicz, A.B. & Read, A.E. (1970) Coeliac infertility: An indication for dietary gluten restriction. *The Lancet* I:412.

Murray, J.A. (2005) Coeliac disease in patients with an affected member, type 1 diabetes, iron deficiency, or osteoporosis? *Gastroenterology* 128(4, Suppl 1):1–9.

Ozaslan, E., Kosenoglu, T. & Kayhan, B. (2004) Coeliac crisis in adults: Report of two cases. *Emergency Medicine* 11:363–365.

Pengiran Tengah, D.S.N.A., Wills, A.J. & Holmes, G.K.T. (2002) Neurological complications of coeliac disease. *Postgraduate Medical Journal* 78:393–398.

Rampertab, S.D., Pooran, N., Brar, P., Sing, P. & Green, P. (2006) Trends in the presentation of celiac disease. *The American Journal of Medicine* 119:355e9–355e14.

Sanders, D.S., Hurlstone, D.P., McAlindon, M.E., Hadjivassiliou, M., Cross, S.S., Wild, G. & Atkins, C.J. (2005) Antibody negative coeliac disease presenting in elderly people – an easily missed diagnosis. *British Medical Journal* 330: 775–776.

Sanders, D.S., Hurlstone, D.P., Stokes, R.O., Rashid, F., Milford-Ward, A., Hadjivassiliou, M. & Lobo, A.J. (2002) Changing face of adult coeliac disease: Experience of a single university hospital in South Yorkshire. *Postgraduate Medical Journal* 78:31–33.

Sanders, D.S., Hurlstone, D.P., McAlindon, M.E., Hadjivassiliou, M., Cross, S.S., Wild, G. & Atkins, C.J. (2005) Antibody negative coeliac disease presenting in elderly people – an easily missed diagnosis. *British Medical Journal* 330:775–776.

Schuppan, D. & Junker, Y. (2007) Turning swords into plowshares: Transglutaminase to detoxify gluten (Editorial). *Gastroenterology* 133(3):1025–1028.

Unsworth, D.J., Lock, E.J. & Harvey, R.F. (1999) Iron deficiency anaemia in premenopausal women. *The Lancet* 353:1100.

Van Der Meer, J.B. (1969) Granular deposits of immunoglobulins in the skin of patients with dermatitis herpetiformis.

An immunofluorescent study. *British Journal of Dermatology* 81:493–503.

Van Heel, D.A. & West, J. (2006) Recent advances in coeliac disease. *Gut* 55:1037–1046.

Ventura, A., Magazzu, G. & Greco, L. (1999) Duration of exposure to gluten and risk for autoimmune disorders in celiac disease. *Gastroenterology* 117:303–310.

Ventura, A., Neri, E., Ughi, C., Leopaldi, A., Citta, A. & Not, T. (2000) Gluten dependent diabetes related and thyroid related autoantibodies in patient with coeliac disease. *Journal of Paediatrics* 137:263.

Walker-Smith, J.A. & Grigor, W. (1969) Coeliac disease in a diabetic child (Letter). *The Lancet* 35:1215–1218.

Walters, J.R.F. (2007) Analysis of the absolute risk in coeliac disease indicates the importance of the prevention of osteoporosis. *Gut* 56(2):310.

Walters, J.R.F. & Van Heel, D.A. (2003) Detecting the risks of osteoporotic fractures in coeliac disease. *Gut* 52(8):1229–1230.

Wilson, J. & Junger, G. (1968) *Principles and Practice of Screening for Disease*. World Health Organization, Geneva.

Winson, L.O., Sano, K., Lebwohl, B., Diamond, B. & Green, P. (2003) Changing presentation of adult coeliac disease. *Digestive Diseases and Sciences* 48(2):395–398.

Zone, J.J. (2005) Skin manifestations of coeliac disease. *Gastroenterology* 128:S87–S91.

Chapter 4
Diagnosing Coeliac Disease

LEARNING OUTCOMES

At the end of this chapter you should be able to:

- Discuss the importance of obtaining an accurate clinical history.
- Describe how to obtain an accurate clinical history.
- Explain the diagnostic pathway including the risks, benefits and alternatives.
- Discuss how nurses can support patients through the diagnostic process.

With the change in disease presentation and the estimation that it remains undiagnosed in 1% of the population (Van Heel & West, 2006), discussion has so far centred on identification of those most at risk of having the disease. What is equally important is ensuring that any diagnosis is made on the basis of sound clinical evidence given the life-long implications of that diagnosis.

Wheat and/or gluten allergies are often self-diagnosed by individuals with a long history of gastrointestinal symptoms. For example, up to 5% of patients with a diagnosis of irritable bowel syndrome (IBS) have coeliac disease (Travis *et al.*, 2005), but along with three quarters of patients with IBS who will never seek medical advice. Nevertheless, finding that a gluten free diet helps their symptoms they will continue to loosely adhere to the diet without the diagnosis that ensures that they receive appropriate education, advice and long-term disease follow-up.

So, before we begin to think about what works in treating illness we need to address the problem 'what's wrong' and this chapter focuses on how nurses might use clinical judgement in this area in taking an accurate history, on autoantibodies as predictors of coeliac disease and on the endoscopic and other diagnostic tools used in obtaining tissue samples.

Once again, although complex, there is a need to understand the pathogenesis of coeliac disease in order to comprehend the significance of both the serological and histopathological results when looking to diagnose the disease. Inaccurate or false test results can cause distress for patients and nurses may well be called upon to explain the significance of findings.

AN ACCURATE HISTORY

Individuals with coeliac disease will attend many different clinics, depending on the presenting symptoms, which as we have seen may range from gastrointestinal to neurological. This section concentrates on taking a general health history regardless of the context of the setting or reason for referral. It is therefore not specific to diagnosing coeliac disease alone. Certainly where there is a high index of suspicion for the disease as with an apparent classic presentation or iron deficiency anaemia, we should be looking closely at family history. History that includes a significant change in nutritional status or bowel habit, infection, recent pregnancy or other autoimmune disorders should arouse suspicion of coeliac disease.

The health history is vital in starting to understand what a person's perception of their health is. It collects mainly subjective data, i.e. what the person says about themselves and very often pinpoints subtle clues that help provide the link to physical examination (deliberately excluded in this section) and subsequent investigation. Yet the history or health interview is often the least well done. Whether in the GP surgery or the outpatient clinic appointment times often dictate the length of time available to take an accurate history, going over medical histories covering decades, which whilst interesting are not always relevant. As important as these are to the individual and to an extent the health interview, without focus and direction important information regarding current health issues is missed, leading to inappropriate investigations and/or delayed diagnoses. 'White coat syndrome' also means individuals may only tell their doctor what they think they want to hear rather than be a burden or appear stupid.

Nurses are often the best placed healthcare professionals to take the health history. Nurse-led clinics will normally have more time devoted to each appointment, giving additional time to form a rapport with the patient. Even out of a clinic environment nurses pick up information through conversation when performing routine tasks and should not underestimate the importance of these conversations. However, these can still be done badly and there are key points to remember in obtaining an accurate history within a clinic setting, some points being equally salient during general conversations.

Opening the interview

How the interview is opened will affect any subsequent dialogue. First impressions are vital when time is limited. If patients have problems accessing hospital facilities, find clinics that are overrunning or are just nervous, these can have a profoundly negative impact on the subsequent interview. Key points to remember are:

- Address the patient by their surname until invited to use their Christian name.
- Apologise if there have been delays, even if they were beyond your control.
- Introduce yourself and your role.
- Clarify the patient's expectation from the visit.
- Set the agenda – Let the patient know the purpose of the interview and the information you are looking to elicit.
- Remember non-verbal behaviour during the interview. Avoid yawning, frowning, slouching, finger tapping, looking at the clock – behaviours that suggest boredom.
- Maintain eye contact with the patient as much as possible.

> **Activity**
>
> Within your clinical area critically analyse the communication between your medical and nursing colleagues and their patients. Where are the similarities and differences in each approach? What are the strengths and weaknesses of each?

Current health problem

This is the data-gathering phase where the interviewer's role is in focusing on the main issues and facilitating appropriate responses. Key points to remember are:

- Start the interview with open-ended questions directed at the major problems but maintaining the focus in time and space, i.e. 'what have been your main symptoms since consulting your doctor?'
- Encourage responses with non-verbal, verbal cues and even silence.
- If you are writing down the patients' response as they are speaking, ask them to continue as a sign that you are listening to what they are saying.
- Clarify responses where there is ambiguity, without being critical of the language the patient uses, i.e. 'can you tell me what you mean by "gastric stomach?"'
- Use what, where and when questions directed to expand on areas of the patient's story and the key characteristics (Table 4.1) of any symptom the patient complains of. Avoid the use of 'why' questions which are often seen to imply disapproval and can make patients defensive.
- Record objectively without interpretation what the patient is saying, using direct quotes where appropriate.
- Summarise the discussion to that point to ensure that you have understood what the patient has said.

Expanding on the initial history

Once the initial information has been gathered the history needs to be expanded on, focusing on reviewing systems and

Table 4.1   Key characteristics of symptoms

1.   Location – Be specific, ask the patient to point to it.
2.   Radiation – Does it spread anywhere else?
3.   Character – What is it like? Encourage descriptive phrases like 'stabbing', 'crushing', 'twisting'.
4.   Severity – Be specific, i.e. on a scale of 1–10.
5.   Duration – How long does it last?
6.   Frequency – How often does it occur? Be specific.
7.   Aggravating factors – What if anything makes it worse?
8.   Relieving factors – What if anything makes it better?
9.   Associated factors – Anything else that contributes to the symptoms?
10.   Effect on daily living – What does it restrict or prevent them from doing?

symptoms that appear to support a particular diagnosis. This needs a degree of both experience and interpretation. Remembering the list of disorders associated with coeliac disease, an open mind is imperative. Key points to remember:

- Be systematic in approach and stay focused, pay attention to the time course of the symptom, has it changed over time?
- Do not forget to note and document the patient's physical appearance (weight, skin pallor, kempt/unkempt).
- Obtain a brief past medical and social history. This should include current medications (including those bought over the counter), surgery, hospitalisations, alcohol/tobacco and drug use, marital and family status, occupation and family history.

Closing the interview

It is important that a patient leaves the interview feeling that they have said all they needed to and have a clear idea as to what will happen next. Key points to remember:

- Draw the interview to a close by asking if there is anything else the patient would like to mention.
- Summarise what you have heard and learnt during the interview.
- Summarise your thoughts about the interview, which will automatically lead on to the next stage of the patients'

management, whether it be investigation or a referral back to the GP. Ensure that the patient leaves knowing why a particular course of action is being taken and how they will be informed of the outcome.

- Where appropriate written information is useful in supporting and clarifying verbal information given. This may be in the form of an information leaflet on a particular test or a patient-centred version of the clinic letter.

Activity

The next time you are assessing a patient think about how you approach the interview. Think about your body language, rapport, questioning style, information giving and the accuracy of the assessment. Invite feedback from your peer group.

SEROLOGICAL SCREENING ANTIBODY TESTS

Where a history leads to a suspicion of coeliac disease, the first step is a serologic test as a non-invasive, cost-effective diagnostic tool. Until a few decades ago, with the perception that the clinical presentation of the disease was consistently gastrointestinal, diagnosis was based on unspecific screening tests aimed at establishing the digestive/absorptive functions of the proximal small intestine, such as faecal fat or glucose tolerance (Fasano & Catassi, 2001). Once it was discovered that the gliadin proteins in wheat were the toxic entities in coeliac disease then came the search to identify the associated antibodies. In simple terms antibodies are produced by the immune system in response to the gliadin proteins that the body perceives to be threatening and are therefore seen in higher than normal levels in individuals with coeliac disease. When there is tissue damage within the mucosa, plasma cells are activated to produce antibodies to gliadin, tissue transglutaminase (tTG) and endomysium, which form the basis of serological tests.

Thanks to this more innovative serological screening the prevalence of coeliac disease and its diverse clinical presentation is becoming increasingly recognised.

Sensitivity and specificity

For any serological test to be effective the techniques have to be refined and well standardised; otherwise there will be inter-laboratory variation in reporting results. So, in looking at the diagnostic performance of the various tests we look at their sensitivity and specificity. Sensitivity is a statistical measure of how well a test correctly identifies a condition; it is the proportion of true positives of all the positive cases in the population. Specificity is a statistical measure of how well a test correctly identifies those that do not have the condition; it is the proportion of true negatives of all the negative cases in the population.

Antigliadin antibody

In 1961, the first clinical studies suggesting antibodies to gluten and other dietary proteins in coeliac disease were published (Taylor *et al.*, 1961). This study showed that antibodies to a pro-teolysed fraction of gluten were significantly higher in both incidence and titre in patients with coeliac disease than in control subjects, with precipitating antibodies found in almost half (44.4%) of patients with idiopathic steatorrhoea compared to 7.8% of controls. Improved methods using the *e*nzyme-*l*inked *i*mmunosorbent *a*ssay (ELISA), a biochemical technique, allowed separation of the immunoglobulin IgA-based and IgG antigliadin antibodies. The sensitivity and specificity of these tests were found to be highly variable. IgG-based tests were generally poor in both parameters whereas the IgA-based test was poorly sensitive but more specific (Hill, 2005) and it is the IgA-based tests that have been more widely developed. The significance of a positive antigliadin antibody is of the non-specific recognition of antibodies leading to mucosal damage as other gastrointestinal disorders are known to induce circulating antigliadin antibodies, including Crohn's disease, food protein intolerance and post-infection malabsorption, leading to the possibility of false-positive results. It is felt that the variability and lower accuracy associated with the antigliadin antibody test now make it unsuitable for screening purposes (Hill, 2005); however, it is useful in children younger than 2 years, as antigliadin antibodies are often present before endomysial antibodies develop in the course of the disease (Burgin-Wolff *et al.*, 1991).

IgA anti-reticulin antibody

Anti-reticulin antibodies were first proposed as a screening test in adult coeliac disease in 1971 (Seah *et al.*, 1971). Sera from coeliac patients were shown to produce a characteristic staining pattern of reticulin fibres in indirect immunofluorescence on sections of rat kidney and liver. Of the five types of reticulin antibodies only one is associated with coeliac disease; it is not very sensitive but it is specific. The overall sensitivity and specificity is difficult to determine as there have been insufficient studies involving the anti-reticulin antibody IgA to provide meaningful data (Hill, 2005). The value of this antibody in screening in clinical practice is therefore felt to be limited.

IgA anti-endomysial antibody

The first reliable screening test was the endomysial antibody (EMA) devised in 1983 by Chorzelski and colleagues. They first reported that sera from patients with dermatitis herpetiformis and coeliac disease reacted with oesophageal substrate from primates. Endomysial antibody is carried out by indirect immunofluorescence on tissue sections from the distal oesophagus of monkeys, which detects antibody activity.

This antibody type has a high sensitivity and specificity identified in early studies (Ferreira *et al.*, 1992) as being 100 and 99% respectively, and in systematic reviews in 2000 and 2005 as 94 and 98% respectively (James & Scott, 2000) and between 86 and 100% sensitivity and 90 and 100% specificity (Hill, 2005).

Despite its high performance there are a number of limitations. Firstly, the EMA serology test is for IgA antibodies, increasing the possibility of false-negative results in those individuals with IgA deficiency. IgA deficiency is found in 2% of coeliac patients and 0.2% of the general population (Lewis & Scott, 2006). A way around this is to test all suspected cases for IgA in addition to EMA or to use IgG-based tests, although these are much less sensitive and specific (AGA, 2006). Another limitation is in the use of monkey oesophagus which incurs both ethical and cost considerations. However, the use of human umbilical cord instead of monkey oesophagus, with no deterioration in assay performance (Ladinser *et al.*, 1994), has provided a cheaper method and does not evoke the ethical concerns encountered when using animals. There is also an American study (Volta *et al.*, 1995), indicating inter-laboratory variation in use of the test, showing a range in sensitivity across six different laboratories from 57 to 90%, although a specificity of 100% for all. This clearly demonstrates the need for standardisation and regulation of laboratory techniques.

Although endomysial antibodies can be used as a monitoring tool in disease follow-up, it is not entirely reliable (The Doctors Laboratory, 2006), but most patients with coeliac disease will be negative for endomysial antibodies after 12–18 months on a gluten free diet.

Tissue transglutaminase antibody

With the limitations of EMA screening and the fact that detecting it using indirect immunofluorescence is time-consuming and operator dependent (AGA, 2006; Fasano & Catassi, 2001) tTG antibody has been investigated as a more reliable alternative.

Tissue transglutaminase is important as it has been identified as the autoantigen in coeliac disease with a unique role in its pathogenesis, able to deamidate or selectively modify gliadin peptides to create new epitopes. An epitope is the part of a macromolecule recognised by the immune system, specifically by antibodies, T cells or B cells. In genetically predisposed individuals these epitopes are recognised by HLA-DQ2 or DQ8 triggering in this case an inflammatory T-cell response and the production of TNF-α and other cytokines to cause mucosal damage (Dieterich *et al.*, 2003).

With the identification of tTG as the autoantigen in coeliac disease an ELISA was developed by Dieterich and colleagues (1998) to assay the tTG antibody titres in coeliac disease. The antigen in the assay has been derived from a number of sources including guinea pig liver, human recombinant (artificial DNA), placenta and red blood cells, and these all have slightly different sensitivities and specificities. In one systematic review comparing the EMA with the tTG (Lewis & Scott, 2006) the EMA test had greater specificity than the that of tTG regardless of whether human umbilicus or monkey oesophagus was used. They also showed that tTG using the human recombinant protein has a greater sensitivity than EMA. The reason for the lower specificity with tTG may be that tTG antibodies to human tissue are also found in patients with severe heart failure, chronic liver disease and primary biliary cirrhosis (Bizzaro *et al.*, 2006; Peracchi *et al.*, 2002; Vecchi *et al.*, 2003). Of interest is that although we discuss serological tests, promising results have been found (Nenna *et al.*, 2005) using tTG antibody testing on saliva both as a screening tool and also in surveillance post-diagnosis.

Tissue transglutaminase IgA antibodies become negative 9–24 months after commencing a gluten free diet (The Doctors Laboratory, 2006) and are a useful and reliable assay in disease monitoring. As with the EMA, the use of tTG antibody is limited in individuals with IgA deficiency as it also tests for IgA antibodies.

HLA-DQ typing

We have already heard that almost all patients with coeliac disease have either the HLA-DQ2 or -DQ8 genotype. However, remembering that they are also found in 40% of the general population (Hourigan, 2006), testing for HLA-DQ2 or -DQ8 is really only useful in saying for certain that a patient does not have coeliac disease in the absence of the relevant DQ allele. Therefore, HLA testing is a useful adjunct only when the diagnosis based on other tests is ambiguous or when testing in the context of disease susceptibility in families (AGA, 2006). It is also important to remember that, as with any other genotyping, resources are available to provide genetic counselling to individuals and their families where required.

Which test?

Serological markers are a cheap and non-invasive method to identify symptomatic and asymptomatic individuals at risk of having coeliac disease in addition to their use in disease follow-up. As has been shown they have different sensitivities and specificities, dependent not only on the commercial test used and its interpretation but also on the geographical and genetic population on which it is used, and therefore should not be used as the sole criterion for making a diagnosis of coeliac disease. The internationally accepted gold standard diagnostic test for coeliac disease remains the demonstration of villous atrophy on duodenal biopsy (Walker-Smith *et al.*, 1990). However, serologic testing for tTG and endomysial antibodies can detect coeliac disease and histopathological examination of endoscopically obtained duodenal biopsies can confirm the diagnosis (AGA, 2006).

Box 4.1 summarises the factors that patients and healthcare professionals need to be aware of as affecting the serological diagnosis of coeliac disease.

Activity

Find out what serological tests are routinely used within your trust to test for coeliac disease? What are strengths and weaknesses of the tests used?

METHODS OF OBTAINING A HISTOLOGICAL DIAGNOSIS

Given the relatively high sensitivity and specificity of serological tests there is some argument as to whether small bowel biopsy is essential for verification of coeliac disease and whether it really is the gold standard diagnostic tool as

Box 4.1 Summary of factors affecting serological-based diagnosis of coeliac disease

1. Two per cent of coeliac patients and 0.2% of the general population are IgA deficient and therefore using IgA-based serology tests in these individuals would be unreliable. IgG-based testing could be considered.
2. There are patients without IgA deficiency who are with negative serology but have positive histology. Therefore, anyone with negative serology in whom there is a strong clinical suspicion of coeliac disease should still undergo endoscopy and duodenal biopsies. Additional tests including IgG-based antibodies or HLA-DQ2/DQ8 assays could be considered.
3. The antigen in the tissue transglutaminase assay has been derived from a number of sources including guinea pig liver, human recombinant, placenta and red blood cells. These all have slightly different sensitivities and specificities.
4. Tissue transglutaminase antibodies to human tissue are also found in patients with severe heart failure, chronic liver disease and primary biliary cirrhosis, with the risk of false-positive results.
5. Gluten restrictions will result in a lowering and subsequent disappearance of all laboratory markers making them useful in disease follow-up; therefore, patients must continue on a gluten-containing diet until a diagnosis is obtained.
6. Testing for HLA-DQ2/DQ8 alleles has a negative predictive value only, but is useful where there is diagnostic ambiguity or for family screening with the availability of genetic counselling services.

internationally recognised (AGA, 2006; BSG, 2002; Walker-Smith *et al.*, 1990).

Some (Rewers, 2005) feel that endoscopy as the gold standard diagnostic tool has its limitations. The mucosal lesions may be patchy and thus missed on biopsy, and in some cases the most severe mucosal changes occur further down the small bowel in the jejunum and are therefore inaccessible to conventional upper gastrointestinal endoscopy. Some (Rondonotti & de Franchis, 2007) also point out that endoscopy is an unpleasant, invasive procedure, which asymptomatic individuals especially may find difficult to contemplate.

However, the diagnostic value of duodenal biopsies is good with a high positive and negative predictive value (Dewar & Ciclitira, 2005), and as there are equally unreliable aspects to serological screening, it is surely better to avoid falsely labelling individuals with a disease that imposes a life-long dietary restriction, by using serological screening to diagnose coeliac disease, and duodenal biopsies to confirm the diagnosis and the histological severity? This provides a complete assessment and a baseline for continued monitoring of those positively identified as having coeliac disease. How we obtain duodenal biopsies has evolved over the years, improving in both accuracy and patient acceptability.

The past – the Crosby–Kugler capsule

Until the 1970s and early 1980s, intestinal biopsies were obtained using metal capsules, perhaps the most widely recognised being the Crosby–Kugler or Crosby capsule, originally invented by Dr William H. Crosby, an American haematologist in 1955 to evaluate coeliac disease in soldiers in Korea. These capsules were attached to a long, thin piece of tubing. Patients were asked to swallow the capsule, with the other end of the tube protruding from the mouth, and then wait for the device to pass into the small intestine; its position was verified by X-ray. Once in the small intestine, suction was applied at the end of the tubing; this would trigger a mechanism in the capsule causing a spring-loaded knife to sweep across an opening in the capsule, cutting away any mucosa which happened to have been sucked into the opening. The capsule was then pulled back up by the tubing and the sample retrieved.

Any nurse who has whiled away her time trying to prime these devices, requiring the manual dexterity, eyesight and patience of a watchmaker and saint combined, will recall just how temperamental they could be, often firing of their own accord before reaching the small intestine or in some cases firing the capsule off of the end of the suction device into the intestine. When successful, the tissue samples they provided were excellent. However, there was no way of gauging their success and the procedure was time-consuming for all concerned. The capsules are still used in certain specialist centres, in particular in diagnosing coeliac disease in children (Dewar & Ciclitira, 2005).

> **Activity**
>
> If you can find a Crosby capsule, have a go at putting it together!

The present – endoscopy

The increased use of endoscopy and reliability of biopsy samples have now largely replaced the use of capsule devices. In addition to the standard upper gastrointestinal endoscopes there are now longer small bowel enteroscopes, which, although not used routinely, do provide a more reliable diagnosis in those patients where it is disputed, as it allows exploration and biopsying further down the small intestine, countering some of the previous arguments (Rewers, 2005) concerning accurate identification of patchy or more distal disease.

Endoscopy is derived from two words – the Greek 'endos' meaning *in* and 'scopeo' meaning to *look*. It encompasses, amongst other procedures, all those that look into the gastrointestinal tract. For patients expecting to undergo an 'endoscopy' it can be confusing to be suddenly faced with information about having an OGD (oesophagogastroduodenoscopy) or gastroscopy in addition to the anxiety engendered by having any procedure that involves somebody pushing a tube down your throat. There is a tendency to use the various terms interchangeably, so it is important that information concerning imminent investigations is given in a clear and concise manner so that patients know the purpose and nature of the test. Clear written information should support any given verbally.

In addition to the standard information given regarding an upper gastrointestinal endoscopy, it is important to ensure that patients continue on a gluten-containing diet until a firm diagnosis has been made. For many, particularly symptomatic patients, it is understandable that they will want to do anything to improve their quality of life and so may exclude gluten from their diet immediately there is a suspicion of a diagnosis of coeliac disease. To avoid wasted or repeat procedures, it is vital to ensure that patients are eating a diet that contains at least 10 g of gluten a day for a minimum 2 weeks prior to the endoscopy. This is equivalent to four slices of bread a day (BSG, 2002).

Current practice is to take endoscopic biopsies from the distal duodenum. If in doubt, these should be repeated, or preferably a jejunal biopsy taken using a small bowel enteroscope (BSG, 2002). Most individuals with coeliac disease will have a small bowel that appears macroscopically normal at endoscopy; however, there are some macroscopic appearances that whilst not diagnostic are associated with a high specificity for the disease when identified. These include more commonly scalloping of the small bowel folds or a mosaic (cracked mud) appearance of the mucosa. Diagnosis relies on the histopathologist's interpretation of the biopsies not on the endoscopist's interpretation of the macroscopic appearances, and patients need to be advised that until these results are known they should continue on a gluten-containing diet.

Upper gastrointestinal endoscopy, as with all endoscopic procedures, is invasive and often unpleasant and not without risk, including haemorrhage, perforation and reaction to the drugs used to perform the procedure. It may need to be repeated either to verify an uncertain diagnosis or to monitor disease outcomes. Therefore, it is important to ensure that the procedure is performed safely and comfortably by a competent endoscopist within a skilled endoscopy team.

Activity

Follow the patient's pathway through an upper gastrointestinal endoscopic procedure. What is the patient's experience? Consider issues such as privacy and dignity, comfort, safety and information giving.

The future – video capsule endoscopy

Although this technique does not involve obtaining duodenal biopsies it is appropriate to discuss this relatively new diagnostic tool at this point.

Over the last few years, video capsule endoscopy (VCE) has been increasingly used in the diagnosis of a variety of small bowel diseases. The initial interest in VCE came from developing a technique that would allow direct visualisation of the entire small intestine to help diagnose obscure gastrointestinal bleeding. More recently, its value as a diagnostic tool in coeliac disease has been highlighted (Culliford *et al.*, 2005; Hopper *et al.*, 2007b; Petroniene *et al.*, 2005). Studies comparing duodenal-biopsy-detected villous atrophy with VCE-detected villous atrophy have shown a positive and negative predictive value for VCE of 100 and 88.0% respectively and a sensitivity and specificity of 85 and 100% respectively (Hopper *et al.*, 2007b).

The VCE device is a sealed capsule powered by on-board batteries, with an imager that takes two photographs at eight times magnification every second. The capsule is activated just prior to use and is swallowed relatively easily by patients with water. It is propelled through the gastrointestinal tract by peristalsis. The images are transmitted in radiofrequency signals to a recording device worn by the patient on a belt around the waist, where they are stored. The battery life of the capsule is around 8 hours, in which time an average 55 000 photographs are taken and stored on the recording device. The capsule passes out of the gut and is not retrieved. The recorder is returned and the images are downloaded onto a computer for viewing.

At this stage, the high cost of VCE means that there are only a small number of centres using the technology and consequently only a small number of patients accessing VCE and an equally small number of operators interpreting the images. Larger patient trials are needed to fully assess the technique in this patient group and as familiarity with the technology is critical in ensuring diagnostic accuracy, inter-observer diagnostic agreement has to be shown, including over the degree of villous atrophy observed. It is, however, an alternative to duodenal biopsy in those patients who refuse or who are unable to undergo upper gastrointestinal endoscopy or in those patients where there is a high suspicion of coeliac disease but negative small bowel histology (Rondonotti & de Franchis, 2007).

PATHOLOGIC ANALYSIS AND DIAGNOSIS

Coeliac disease is characterised histologically by loss of the normal villous structure in the small intestine with various degrees of villous atrophy (a lowering of the villous height to crypt depth ratio), an increase in epithelial lymphocytes and extensive surface cell damage and infiltration of the lamina propria with inflammatory cells (Bardella *et al.*, 2007).

When analysing duodenal biopsies the histopathologist will be reliant on the information sent with the samples to accurately interpret them. As a rule, four samples should be taken to ensure that patchy changes are less likely to be missed. They should be labelled clearly to state where they have been taken from and include relevant clinical information such as:

- Is there positive serology or HLA-DQ assay?
- Is there a family history of coeliac disease?
- Has the patient been eating a gluten-containing diet, i.e. is this part of a gluten challenge?
- Has the patient had previous duodenal biopsies taken?
- Were the biopsies taken diagnostic or to check for mucosal recovery?

The Marsh (Marsh, 1992) classification has been widely adopted to describe the progression of mucosal abnormalities seen in individuals with coeliac disease (see Figure 4.1 and Table 4.2).

As with the clinical presentation of coeliac disease there is increasing recognition that the pathological presentation of the disease also varies. Conventionally, a diagnosis of coeliac disease was made on the basis of a histological abnormality equivalent to a Marsh 3 lesion (Dewar & Ciclitira, 2005). There are, however, studies showing individuals with Marsh 1 and 2 type lesions, i.e. without villous atrophy, whose histological abnormalities improve on a gluten free diet (Tursi & Brandimarte, 2003). Although Marsh (1992) suggests that type 1 and 2 lesions are the first stages of a gradual derangement in the intestinal mucosa in coeliac patients, there are a number of difficulties shown with diagnosing coeliac disease on the basis of these lesions (Dewar & Ciclitira, 2005). One is that there is poor

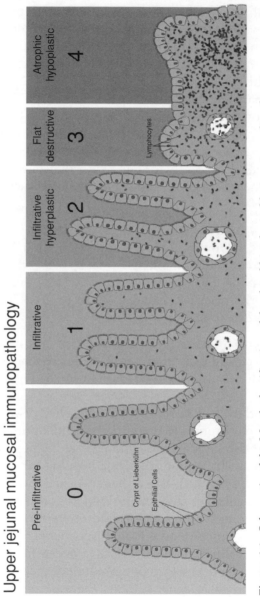

Upper jejunal mucosal immunopathology

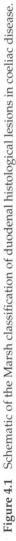

Figure 4.1   Schematic of the Marsh classification of duodenal histological lesions in coeliac disease.

Table 4.2   The Marsh classification of duodenal histological lesions in coeliac disease

Histological type	Intraepithelial lymphocytes	Glandular crypts	Villous architecture
0	Normal	Normal	Normal
1	Increased	Normal	Normal
2	Increased	Hyperplastic	Normal
3a	Increased	Hyperplastic	Partial atrophy
3b	Increased	Hyperplastic	Subtotal atrophy
3c	Increased	Hyperplastic	Total atrophy
4	Increased	Hypoplastic	Flat

inter-observer correlation in interpreting Marsh 1 lesions. The second is that we do not know whether individuals without villous atrophy have the same adverse health risks as the traditional coeliac patient with villous atrophy and thirdly that the morbidity data available at the current time have been obtained largely from symptomatic patients diagnosed with villous atrophy. Clearly as recognised by some (Dewar & Ciclitira, 2005), it is sensible to advise a gluten free diet in those individuals who have symptoms or clinical manifestations suggestive of coeliac disease; however, it may be difficult to persuade individuals without such symptoms or manifestations to follow a gluten free diet on the basis of a 'possibility' that they have the disease. It also means that if Marsh 1 and 2 lesions are considered to represent active coeliac disease requiring a gluten free diet then normalisation after gluten withdrawal will need to be histologically confirmed in all cases, knowing that the intestinal mucosa may improve but does not normalise in all coeliac patients even where clinical remission is achieved (Bardella *et al.*, 2007). This is more difficult to assess in the absence of villous atrophy and so could be distressing for patients who might feel that their adherence to the diet is in question or worry that they are at risk of eventual complications from continued mucosal damage.

Marsh 4 lesions are a rare histologic finding thought to signify irreversible injury caused by chronic inflammation, related to refractory coeliac disease and the development of enteropathy-associated T-cell lymphoma (Dewar & Ciclitira, 2005). These patients need specialist advice and follow-up.

Activity

Look at the histology reports of any coeliac patients in your care. What is the Marsh classification or, if not stated, the degree of villous atrophy? Match this to their presenting symptoms. Is there a link between the severity of their symptoms and the degree of mucosal damage?

Towards a definitive diagnosis

This chapter has highlighted the importance of accurately identifying those individuals who may have coeliac disease, which is achieved to begin with by obtaining an accurate history, in which nurses may or may not play a significant role. Where serological and/or histological diagnosis is concerned, we have seen that whilst the various diagnostic tools have an impressive sensitivity and specificity there are drawbacks to all, which may result in false-positive or false-negative outcomes if used injudiciously or in the wrong combination. Results are not always straightforward and studies are being undertaken (Hopper *et al.*, 2007a) to evaluate clinical decision tools, which aim to amalgamate the most sensitive and specific of the tests in the most effective way to maximise the accurate detection of coeliac disease.

How these tests are interpreted is best left to the relevant experts. However, nurses have a pivotal role to play in guiding patients through the diagnostic quagmire, providing information, education and support through the various procedures and tests. For some asymptomatic patients the diagnosis may be sudden and unexpected, whilst equally for some symptomatic patients the diagnosis may remain elusive. Support at this stage helps patients to come to terms and accept the diagnosis of what is a life-long chronic disease and dauntingly a life-long gluten free diet. This undoubtedly leads to much better conformity with treatment and management and hopefully therefore better health outcomes.

HINTS AND TIPS

- Sit in on consultations with medical colleagues to observe the medical assessment process.
- Map out the diagnostic pathway and familiarise yourself with the processes and procedures. Visit the departments, i.e. endoscopy and pathology, to improve your understanding of the patient's experience.
- Discuss with your medical colleagues how they envisage the service looking. At what phase along the pathway will you become directly involved in patient care?
- Use this information to write out a business case for the service. (Your trust will have a template for this.) This is essential to ensure that the service is supported. Make certain that all service providers are acknowledged and involved in the start-up process and that communication with all concerned remains effective and efficient.

REFERENCES

American Gastroenterological Association (2006) AGA Institute Medical Position Statement on the diagnosis and management of coeliac disease. *Gastroenterology* 131:1977–1980.

Bardella, M.T., Velio, P., Cesana, B.M., Prampolini, L., Casella, G., Di Bella, C., Lanzini, A., Gambarotti, M., Bassotti, G. & Villanacci, V. (2007) Coeliac disease: A histological follow-up study. *Histopathology* 50:465–471.

Bizzaro, N., Tampoia, M., Villalta, D., Platzgummer, S., Liguori, M., Tozzoli, R. & Tonutti, E. (2006) Low specificity of anti-tissue transglutaminase antibodies in patients with primary biliary cirrhosis. *Journal of Clinical Laboratory Analysis* 20:184–189.

British Society of Gastroenterology (2002) *Guidelines for the Management of Patients with Coeliac Disease.* BSG, London.

Burgin-Wolff, A., Gaze, H., Hadziselimovic, F., Huber, H., Lentze, M.J., Nussle, D. & Reymond-Berthet, C. (1991) Antigliadin and antiendomysium antibody determination for coeliac disease. *Archives of Disease in Childhood* 66:941–947.

Chorzelski, T.P., Sulej, T., Tchorzewski, H., Jablonska, S., Beutner, G.H. & Kumar, V. (1983) IgA class endomysium antibodies in dermatitis herpetiformis and coeliac disease. *Annals of the New York Academy of Sciences* 420:325–334.

Culliford, A., Daly, J., Diamond, B., Moshe, R. & Green, P.H.R. (2005) The value of wireless capsule endoscopy in patients with complicated coeliac disease. *Gastrointestinal Endoscopy* 62:55–61.

Dewar, D.H. & Ciclitira, P.J. (2005) Clinical features and diagnosis of coeliac disease. *Gastroenterology* 128:S19–S24.

Dieterich, W., Laag, E., Schopper, H., Volta, U., Feruguson, A., Gillet, H., Riecken, E.O. & Schuppan, D. (1998) Antibodies to tissue transglutaminase as predictors of coeliac disease. *Gastroenterology* 115(6):1317–1321.

Dieterich, W., Trapp, D., Esslinger, B., Leidenberger, M., Hahn, H., Schuppan, D. & Piper, J. (2003) Autoantibodies of patients with coeliac disease are insufficient to block tissue transglutaminase activity. *Gut* 52(11):1562–1566.

Fasano, A. & Catassi, C. (2001) Current approaches to diagnosis and treatment of coeliac disease: An evolving spectrum. *Gastroenterology* 120:636–651.

Ferreira, M., Lloyd, D.S., Butler, M., Scott, D., Clark, M. & Kumar, P. (1992) Endomysial antibody: Is it the best screening test for coeliac disease? *Gut* 33:1633–1637.

Hill, I.D. (2005) What are the sensitivity and specificity of serologic tests for coeliac disease? Do sensitivity and specificity vary in different populations? *Gastroenterology* 128:S25–S32.

Hopper, A.D., Cross, S.S., Hurlstone, D.P., McAlindon, M.E., Lobo, A.J., Hadjivassiliou, M., Sloan, M.E., Dixon, S. & Sanders, D.S. (2007a) Pre-endoscopy serological testing for coeliac disease: Evaluation of a clinical decision tool. *British Medical Journal* 334:729–734.

Hopper, A.D., Sidhu, R., Hurlstone, D.P., McAlindon, M.E. & Sanders, D.S. (2007b) Capsule endoscopy: An alternative to duodenal biopsy for the recognition of villous atrophy in coeliac disease? *Digestive and Liver Disease* 39:140–145.

Hourigan, C.S. (2006) The molecular basis of coeliac disease. *Clinical and Experimental Medicine* 6:53–59.

James, M.W. & Scott, B.B. (2000) Endomysial antibody in the diagnosis and management of coeliac disease. *Postgraduate Medical Journal* 76:466–468.

Ladinser, B., Rossipal, E. & Pittschielder, K. (1994) Endomysium antibodies in coeliac disease: An improved method. *Gut* 35:76–778.

Lewis, N.R. & Scott, B.B. (2006) Systematic review: The use of serology to exclude or diagnose coeliac disease (a comparison of endomysial and tissue transglutaminase antibody tests). *Alimentary Pharmacology and Therapeutics* 24:47–54.

Marsh, M. (1992). Gluten major histocompatability complex and the small intestine. A molecular and immunologic approach to the spectrum of gluten sensitivity. *Gastroenterology* 102(1):330–354.

Nenna, R., Tiberti, C., Mura, S., Ferri, M., Thanasi, E., Luparia, R., Castronovo, A., Fiore, B., Verrienti, A. & Bonamico, M. (2005) The role of salivary anti-transglutaminase autoantibodies at the diagnosis and follow-up of coeliac disease. *Pediatric Research* 52(2):399.

Peracchi, M., Trovato, C., Longhi, M., Gasparin, M., Conte, D., Tarantino, C., Prati, D. & Bardella, M.T. (2002) Tissue transglutaminase antibodies in patients with end-stage heart failure. *American Journal of Gastroenterology* 97(11):2850–2854.

Petroniene, R., Dubcenco, E., Baker, J., Ottaway, C., Tang, S., Zanti, S., Streutker, C., Gardiner, G., Warren, R. & Jeejeebhoy, K. (2005) Given® Capsule endoscopy in coeliac disease: Evaluation of diagnostic accuracy and interobserver agreement. *American Journal of Gastroenterology* 100:685–694.

Rewers, M. (2005) Epidemiology of coeliac disease: What are the prevalence, incidence and progression of coeliac disease? *Gastroenterology* 128:S47–S51.

Rondonotti, E. & de Franchis, R. (2007) Commentary-diagnosing coeliac disease: Is the videocapsule a suitable tool? *Digestive and Liver Disease* 39(2):140–145.

Seah, PP., Fry, L., Hoffbrand, A.V. & Holborrow, E.J. (1971) Tissue antibodies in dermatitis herpetiformis and adult coeliac disease. *The Lancet* 1:834–836.

Taylor, K.B., Thomson, D.L., Truelove, S.C. & Wright, R. (1961) An immunological study of coeliac disease and idiopathic steatorrhoea. *British Medical Journal* 2:1727–1731.

The Doctors Laboratory (2006) Coeliac genotyping. TDL Pathology Website. http://www.tdlpathology.com/index.php?option=com_content&task=view&id=36&Itemi. Accessed 9 March 2007.

Travis, S.P.L., Ahmad, T., Collier, J. & Steinhart, A.H. (2005) Irritable bowel syndrome. In *Pocket Consultant Gastroenterology.* Blackwell Publishing, Oxford, pp. 335–345.

Tursi, A. & Brandimarte, G. (2003) The symptomatic and histologic response to a gluten free diet in patients with borderline enteropathy. *Journal of Clinical Gastroenterology* 36:13–17.

Van Heel, D.A. & West, J. (2006) Recent advances in coeliac disease. *Gut* 55:1037–1046.

Vecchi, M., Folli, C., Donato, M.F., Formenti, S., Arosio, E. & De Franchis, R. (2003) High rate of positive anti-tissue transglutaminase antibodies in chronic liver disease: Role of liver decompensation and of the antigen source. *Scandinavian Journal of Gastroenterology* 38:50–54.

Volta, U., Molinaro, N., De Franceschi, L., Fratangelo, D. & Bianchi, F.B. (1995) IgA anti-endomysial antibodies on human umbilical cord tissue for coeliac disease screening. Save both money and monkeys. *Digestive Disease Science* 40:1902–1905.

Walker-Smith, J.A., Guandalini, S., Schmitz, J., Shmerling, D.H. & Visakorpi, J.K. (1990) Revised criteria for diagnosis of coeliac disease (report of the Working Group of European Society of Paediatric Gastroenterology and Nutrition). *Archives of Disease in Childhood* 65:909–911.

Chapter 5
The Treatment of Coeliac Disease

LEARNING OUTCOMES

At the end of this chapter you should be able to:

- Discuss the importance of the gluten free diet as the cornerstone of treatment.
- Describe what a gluten free diet is.
- Discuss the nutritional needs of coeliac patients including the implications of balancing this with other diets and/or food allergies.
- Discuss the strengths and limitations of the codes of practice aimed at protecting the coeliac patient as a consumer.
- Discuss food labelling and the implications for coeliac patients.
- Discuss the support needed to comply with treatment.

When this chapter was first drafted its title was 'Dietary Treatment'; however, this seemed to imply that there were other treatment options. The gluten free diet or, as perhaps more aptly termed by some (Kupper, 2005) medical nutrition therapy, is the only accepted treatment of coeliac disease. As such it is vital that patients receive the appropriate education, motivation and support to achieve and maintain this life-long treatment and nurses have a key role to play in all of these areas, alongside the dietitian, whose role is pivotal.

This chapter discusses diet as the cornerstone of treatment, discussing how to avoid the inevitable traps when trying to shop, cook and eat without gluten whilst balancing family and professional commitments. It also shows how internationally work is being undertaken to ensure a high level of consumer protection and fair practice in the trade of food and agricultural products that claim to be gluten free.

THE GLUTEN FREE DIET

The gluten free diet excludes the disease-activating storage proteins (prolamins) gliadin, hordein, secalin and avenin, found in wheat, barley, rye and oats, respectively. As we know it is these proteins that activate the particular immune response that causes damage to the intestinal mucosa, with resultant inflammation releasing cytokines and other inflammatory mediators. The presence of gluten in the diet of those individuals with coeliac disease leads to self-perpetuating mucosal damage, whereas removal of gluten from the diet results in full mucosal recovery (Fasano & Cattasi, 2001) and avoidance of the risks associated with continued exposure to gluten, including small bowel cancers. Therefore, the only treatment that can be recommended currently for coeliac disease is a strict, life-long gluten free diet, irrespective of the severity of the symptoms, something that asymptomatic patients find hard to comprehend initially. Hence, selling it as a form of medication can be useful. Some patients and healthcare professionals even today still think that you grow out of the disease, a theory that needs to be dispelled early on.

Symptomatic and clinical improvements can be seen within the first few weeks of a gluten free diet; however, full restoration of intestinal mucosa may take up to 2 years, depending on the extent and severity of the initial damage (Danowski *et al.*, 2003).

Whilst the focus of nutrition therapy in coeliac disease has a tendency to be around those foods allowed and not allowed in a gluten free diet, it is important to remember the overall nutritional quality of the diet, taking into consideration, in addition to iron, calcium and fibre intake, other food aversions, allergies or intolerances that could lead to a gluten free but nutritionally inadequate diet (Shepherd & Gibson, 2006; Thompson *et al.*, 2005). For example, some coeliac patients will suffer with lactose intolerance, because the damage to the small intestine prevents the production of sufficient quantities of lactase, the digestive enzyme essential for the complete digestion and absorption of lactose. Similar symptoms may arise from an intolerance to other carbohydrates such as sucrose and lactulose, but lactose is particularly important in coeliac patients as the chief source of lactose in, dairy products, and is also the chief source of calcium, necessary for maintaining bone health. This is why the role of the dietitian is crucial not only in having the expertise to educate the individual on the role of gluten in the diet but in assessing current nutritional deficiencies or problem areas and ensuring that they maintain an overall nutritionally balanced diet. However, many patients are not referred to a dietitian especially in the United States (Case, 2005) where, although it is seen as a priority, there is a limited or total lack of reimbursement for nutrition therapy and education by insurance companies. This leaves many patients paying for the service and therefore marginalises those unable or less willing to pay for treatment advice.

Activity

What is the role of the dietitians within your clinical area in supporting patients with coeliac disease? What information, advice and support do they provide?

What is in a gluten free diet?

In order to understand what a gluten free diet consists of we need to start with the very basic storage proteins and what seeds, grains and starches contain gluten and which do not (see Table 5.1). These form the basic ingredients of gluten free foods. As can be seen, some of the hybrid seeds and grains listed are relatively unfamiliar and not readily available in the high street. Even with apparently straightforward foods confusion can arise when faced with labelling that includes the word 'flour' as some assume that flour automatically contains gluten forgetting that rice flour, maize flour, potato flour etc. are in fact gluten free. Couscous contains gluten, whilst buckwheat does

Table 5.1 Grains, seeds and other starch sources classified according to whether gluten free or not

Allowed in a gluten free diet	Not allowed in a gluten free diet
Amaranth grain	Wheat (including wheat starch)
Arrowroot	Barley (and malt extracts)
Buckwheat	Couscous (wheat and barley)
Corn/maize	Rye
Mesquite seed pod (North American)	Spelt
Millet	Triticale seed
Quinoa grain (South American)	Kamut grain
Rice – all rice types	Oats
Sorghum grain (Milo)	
Soy	
Tapioca	

not. Cornflour is gluten free only if it is pure maize flour as there is a wheaten cornflour. Wheat starch would appear to be contradictory but is accepted in a gluten free diet in some European countries if labelled Codex wheat starch but should be avoided if simply labelled wheat starch; if listed simply as modified starch without stating its source (i.e. wheat) then it has to be gluten free. Even if a product contains apparently gluten free seeds or grains, there is still the risk of cross-contamination during production, which has led to much of the issue around including oats in the diet as oat products carry a high risk of contamination from other cereals.

Confused? – Is it any wonder patients are.

If those with coeliac disease are to stand any hope of life-long compliance to a gluten free diet, they need to feel confident and competent in choosing the right foods. Broadly speaking, there are three types of food that they need to consider (Shepherd & Gibson, 2006), and we will look as to how that translates into shopping for gluten free foods a little further on. These groups are:

1. Foods that are totally gluten free in their natural state and have not gone through any manufacturing process, fresh fruit, vegetables, meat, fish, milk, eggs etc.
2. Foods clearly labelled as gluten free, which means that they have to comply, as a minimum, with the Codex standard

(see below); these include the gluten free foods available on prescription.
3. Foods not labelled as gluten free but which may still be suitable for a gluten free diet by interpreting the gluten status of each individual ingredient within the total product.

Thankfully, as most coeliac patients tell us, dietary treatments have improved significantly over the last decade. However, with the rise in the international food trade and the amount of processed foods including ready meals, shopping for all but natural unprocessed foods can be a nightmare. Standards and codes of practice restrict the amount of gluten allowed in gluten free products and aim to ensure clearer labelling, and so it is useful to make certain that new coeliac patients are made aware of the Codex standard and labelling laws that aim to protect them as consumers.

The Codex standard

The Codex Alimentarius Commission was created in 1963 by the Food and Agriculture Organization (FAO) and the World Health Organization (WHO), to develop food standards, guidelines and codes of practice. It deals with the management of production processes and the operation of government regulatory systems for food safety and consumer protection including food labelling, additives and contaminants. Membership is open to all member nations and associate members of FAO/WHO, currently comprising over 160 countries. The Food Standards Agency represents the United Kingdom at Codex.

Codex standards are developed through a formal procedure consisting of eight stages or steps which rely on consensus for agreement. A vote from all member countries can be called if consensus is not achieved but this is avoided where possible. What is interesting is that agreed standards are voluntary; however, with the increase in the international food trade and consumer concern around food safety and quality these standards have become the accepted reference documents for all those engaged in consumer protection.

Box 5.1 Principles of Codex Standard 118 for gluten free foods

---

1. The standard applies to those processed foods which have been prepared especially to meet the dietary needs of persons intolerant to gluten.
2. It does not apply to foods which in their natural form do not contain gluten.
3. Gluten is defined as those proteins normally found in wheat, triticale, rye, barley and oats.
4. A gluten free food consists of those foods containing gluten which have been processed to render them gluten free or in which the ingredients normally present containing gluten have been substituted for ingredients not containing gluten. Or where the product contains a mixture of the two.
5. Gluten free means that the total nitrogen content of gluten-containing cereal grains should not exceed 0.05 g per 100 g of dry product, or 0.3% protein.
6. Gluten free foods must supply approximately the same amount of vitamins and minerals as the original foods they replace, in line with each country's own legislation.
7. In addition to general labelling standards, the term *gluten free* must appear on the product label in immediate proximity to the product name.

The Codex Alimentarius Standard was used worldwide to set the standards of gluten content allowed in a food product to be considered gluten free for international trade. Up until recently, they defined 'gluten free' as foods containing <0.3% (200 parts per million, ppm) protein from a grain containing gluten, defined as wheat, triticale, rye, barley and oats. Box 5.1 outlines the principles of the standard, which it is important to understand. However, this standard was first adopted by the Codex Commission in 1976 and amended in 1983 (Codex Alimentarius Commission, 1981, Standard 118) since which time methods used to measure gluten levels in foods have become so sensitive that they can detect a concentration of 2–5 ppm, over 500 times more sensitive than the Codex standard (Shepherd & Gibson, 2006).

Worldwide there remained no agreement on just how much gluten a person with coeliac disease could tolerate. The Codex definition came under review in the 1990s and remained until recently at step seven whilst the committee evaluated further scientific research and clarification on tolerance levels, in addition to clarification of the best methods of detecting gluten. They evaluated a system called R5-ELISA which is able to identify the relevant prolamines with a detection limit of 3.2 ppm gluten (Valdes *et al.*, 2003). There had also been estimates made on the safe threshold for daily gluten intake (Collin *et al.*, 2004) of 100 ppm gluten (100 mg gluten/kg). Which was half that recommended in the current Codex standard. This study took into consideration the residual gluten found in the so-called gluten free products and the mucosal recovery of those following a diet within the stipulated threshold. There were also smaller studies (Catassi *et al.*, 2007) suggesting that the safe threshold for daily gluten intake should be even lower, not exceeding 50 ppm gluten (50 mg gluten/kg), a quarter of that recommended in the current Codex standard. As this goes to press the Codex review has finally reached stage eight and the Codex standard for gluten free labelling has been lowered to 20 mg/kg or 20 ppm (coeliac.org.uk, 2008). The new standard will be called the 'codex standard for foods for special dietary use for persons intolerant to gluten' and when adopted will create two standards for gluten free foods.

- Specially manufactured products with a gluten level of less than 20 ppm or 20 mg/kg can be labelled as 'gluten free'
- Specially manufactured products that have a gluten level higher than 20 mg/kg but lower than 100 mg/kg will still be available but cannot be labelled as 'gluten free'.

Straightforward, I am afraid not. Remembering that the Codex standard is voluntary, the debate into safe thresholds has led to other countries adopting their own standards in defining what constitutes a gluten free food. Whilst many European countries followed the old Codex standard and will undoubtedly follow the new, Canada and parts of the United States must meet standards that state that a product cannot be labelled 'gluten free' unless it does not contain any wheat, including spelt, kamut, oats, barley, triticale, rye or part thereof, whether or not it is gluten free on a sensitive assay such as the R5-ELISA (Canadian Food Inspection Agency, 2003; Coeliac Sprue Association). In other words, it must only contain naturally gluten free grains as highlighted in Table 5.1. Meanwhile, parts of New Zealand and Australia do permit the inclusion of gluten free wheat-derived products but with much stricter standards, in that foods labelled gluten free must have no ingredient containing detectable gluten (<10 ppm) (Shepherd & Gibson, 2006).

What is clear is that a label stating 'gluten free' can mean a number of things depending on its country of origin but does not always mean the complete absence of those proteins commonly found in wheat, barley, oats and rye and their hybrids. Given the sensitivity to gluten of some individuals with coeliac disease, this could be of considerable importance when looking to achieve complete mucosal healing and control of symptoms, especially for those with more classic presentations of the disease. It does, however, present a minefield when trying to provide appropriate education and support without engendering a sense of fear each time individuals with coeliac disease walk into a food store. Understanding food labels is obviously crucial, but just how easy is it?

Understanding labelling rules

Being able to read and interpret food labels could be thought of as essential skills for those with coeliac disease? Although support organizations provide updated directories on those products that are deemed 'safe' to include in a gluten free diet, in the long-term they should be used as support rather than relied on as the only source of information, as most coeliac patients will not want to walk round with a food directory permanently in their back pocket. It is about adopting a lifestyle of constant vigilance, which is not easy in practice, made worse by the fact that not only is there no universal agreement on permissible gluten levels in food but there is also no universal legislation requiring the complete labelling of ingredients contained in processed foods.

The law on food labelling is complex and amended frequently as you would expect in a rapidly changing and expanding food market. Furthermore, it does not provide an authoritative statement or interpretation of the law and can only be interpreted through the courts. So, although the term 'law' is frequently applied, until tested in court it is guidance only. However, manufacturers would be wise to show adoption of these measures, so that if they are required to defend their practice in law they can show defence of due diligence. Certainly, it is thought that adoption of these measures in the United Kingdom will negate against additional legislation with regard to precautionary labelling (Mills *et al.*, 2004).

In addition to criminal liability, manufacturers can be prosecuted under civil law either under the product liability provision of the Consumer Protection Act (Her Majesty's Stationery Office, 1987) or under the common law of negligence.

In the United Kingdom, one element of the Food Standards Agency (FSA)'s role is to help to prevent the inaccurate labelling or description of foods which, although not necessarily harmful, when done deliberately may constitute fraud. The two main acts that can be applied to food safety are the Trade Descriptions Act (1968), which makes it an offence to apply a false trade description to any goods, and the Food Safety Act (1990), which makes it an offence to sell food for human consumption that:

- Is injurious to health.
- Fails to comply with food safety requirements.
- Is falsely described, labelled or advertised for sale.
- Is not of the nature, substance or quality demanded by the end consumer.

Within the Food Safety Act (1990), there are the food labelling regulations (Her Majesty's Stationary Office, 1996), which in themselves are complex but give information on the basic labelling requirements. One useful reference document is the *Guidance on Allergen Management and Consumer Information* (FSA, 2006). This document gives the current statutory ingredients listing on the 12 most common European food allergens, which include gluten, as per the European labelling directive (European Union Labelling Directive, 2003/89/EC) (Box 5.2). Remembering that it provides guidance only, the European Union document gives a risk-based approach as to the appropriate use of label statements to advise consumers with food allergies, incorporating European legislation that advises manufacturers that where the specified allergenic foods or their derivatives are used as ingredients in pre-packed foods it is

Box 5.2 Current allergens listed in European labelling legislation (taken from FSA, 2006)

1. Cereals containing gluten
2. Crustaceans
3. Egg
4. Fish
5. Peanuts
6. Milk
7. Nuts
8. Soya
9. Sesame
10. Celery
11. Mustard
12. Sulphur dioxide and sulphites

indicated on the labelling. It must be indicated within the ingredients; a separate allergy advice box is often used but is only a recommendation so that patients should know to always check ingredients listings in the absence of any other labelling. From 25 November 2005, products not complying with this European legislation were prohibited. It has also meant the abolition of the 25% rule, which stated that labels did not need to list individual ingredients if they were part of a compound ingredient and if the compound ingredient made up less than 25% of the product.

This legislation does not cover allergens that are unintentionally present as a result of cross-contamination. The Food Standards Agency (2006) document gives guidance to manufacturers through the good manufacturing practices (GMPs) regarding managing the risk of cross-contamination. GMP controls have a commitment to ensuring that products meet food safety, quality and legal requirements. It is helpful to note the Food Standard Agency's listing of the possible sources of cross-contamination (FSA, 2006) as most of these can be applied outside of the food industry as considerations by individuals with coeliac disease particularly when dining out (see Figure 5.1).

Below are just some of the labelling that you might find on packaged food products.

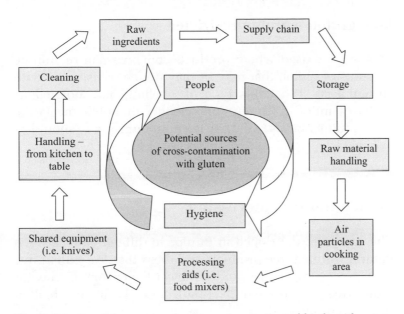

Figure 5.1   Possible sources of cross-contamination of foods with potential allergens. (Adapted from *Potential sources of cross contamination*, FSA, 2006, p. 13.)

Gluten free

Labelling laws state that a product can be labelled 'free from' only if it has been tested for traces of the potential allergen. Therefore, although it sounds like an absolute claim, the only scientific claim in most countries is that samples of the product were shown to be below the analytical limit of detection of a testing method on one or more occasion. In the United States, Canada and Australia, gluten free refers to a food item or ingredient that is 100% gluten free, zero tolerance being the strictest interpretation.

Naturally gluten free

This term was developed by the European coeliac community for products that occur in nature without gluten, i.e. contain those non-gluten-containing seeds and grains as mentioned in Table 5.1.

Low gluten – gluten restricted

This term is used where products contain small or minute amounts of gluten that may or may not be measurable with current tests. What this type of labelling may not tell us is the quantity of gluten and whether or not it meets the Codex Alimentarius Standard as a minimum and so should be avoided.

Gluten free – in processing

This term was developed in Europe to differentiate between naturally gluten free products and those that test gluten free after processing. These products meet the current Codex for gluten free (0.3% protein, 200 ppm), but will change in light of the revised standard.

'May contain' gluten

Some labels say 'may' contain gluten, which means that even though no gluten has been intentionally added, the manufacturer cannot guarantee that gluten has not accidentally got into the product. This type of labelling covers cross-contamination and is particularly important to those with potentially fatal allergies such as nut allergies.

Gluten is often present in food as a hidden ingredient (Lee, 2005). Surveys (Zarkadas *et al.*, 2006) show that up to 83% of coeliac patients find difficulty in finding gluten free foods. Despite labelling regulations, coeliac patients therefore need to become expert label readers. No matter how familiar individuals may feel with a particular brand of food, product formulations can and do change and ingredient lists must be checked each time the product is purchased.

So, how do those with coeliac disease avoid the pitfalls, when faced day to day with nutritionally supporting both themselves and their extended family, with often limited budgets and time?

AVOIDING THE TRAPS – SHOPPING, COOKING AND EATING WITHOUT GLUTEN

Part of the education and support of patients when diagnosed with coeliac disease is in helping patients to feel confident that what they are eating is gluten free. Engendering a sense of fear or giving dogmatic advice at the outset will only lead to demotivation and poor compliance.

The importance of dietetic support cannot be stressed as providing expert assessment, advice and guidance at the outset, but nursing support should continue alongside and beyond those visits.

For many individuals a diagnosis of coeliac disease can result in almost a grief reaction, beginning with a phase of shock or disbelief through to a phase of anguish and possibly difficulty in planning the future but eventually leading to a phase of resolution. At diagnosis, it is acceptable to tell patients that they will make mistakes and that what is a fairly radical change in lifestyle will take time to adjust to and result initially in trial and error. In addition to advice as to what constitutes a gluten free food, they need practical advice to help them when buying and cooking foods, eating out and travelling. The key message here is 'If in doubt – leave it out' and then seek advice from the food manufacturer, national/local coeliac group or healthcare professional.

Shopping lists

Once individual nutritional needs have been assessed by a dietitian, an easy way to start is to look at making three shopping lists. As individuals become confident with the format of these lists they will find it easier to identify the foods where more vigilance is required when shopping.

The first list consists of those products which in their natural state (i.e. raw, uncooked and unprocessed) are totally gluten free. These include fresh fruit, vegetables, eggs, milk and meat. Caution should be exercised however where raw meats have been pre-packed, to ensure that they have not been coated with any seasonings including seasoned salts that contain gluten, or are prepared with a stuffing, as simply removing the stuffing will not remove the gluten.

Activity

Try shopping as a coeliac patient. Look at the packaging to interpret the gluten status of the foods on your shopping list. How easy or difficult did you find it? How far round the store did you get before you gave up!

The second list should consist of prescription foods. The dietary exclusion of gluten is a treatment and not a diet that individuals would choose and as we have already seen it is important to ensure that the diet is balanced in terms of meeting essential nutritional requirements, often already lacking at diagnosis because of the associated malabsorption. Many of the foods excluded are basic staple foods like bread. Not only are many of these gluten free foods not widely available, especially in rural areas, but their cost can be astronomical, with a loaf of bread half the size but costing up to three times as much as its gluten-containing counterpart. In the United Kingdom as in many countries staple foods are available on prescription, to encourage compliance with a healthy balanced diet. Gluten free prescribable items are given a unit value based on their carbohydrate and energy content and their cost (Table 5.2).

Table 5.2 Units represented by the prescribable gluten free food item

Prescribable food item	Unit
400 g bread	1
400 g rolls/baguettes	1
500 g bread mix/flour mix/pastry mix/cake mix	2
100 g sweet/savoury biscuits/crackers	$^1/_2$
150 g sweet/savoury biscuits/crackers	$^3/_4$
200 g sweet/savoury biscuits/crackers/crisp breads	1
250 g pasta	1
500 g pasta	2
2 × 110 g − 180 g pizza bases	1

Blow *et al.*, 2005, p. 11, reproduced with permission from Hilary Franklin Healthcare Communications.

Initially, it can be quite difficult to estimate how much is required; a useful starting point is to get individuals to write a list of the bread, pasta, cakes, biscuits, pastries and flour they consumed in a month before they first experienced symptoms (Blow *et al.*, 2005). This can then be used to work out the foods required against what is available on prescription (Table 5.3). Each prescription, and hence shopping list, should be for a month's worth of food. Prescribable foods tend to have a shorter shelf life and therefore it is important not to over stock. It is also essential to take into consideration individual preference and choice. In the same way as shoppers would walk into a supermarket and choose a loaf of bread, so shoppers with coeliac disease should be able to exercise some choice over the food available to them on prescription and alter that prescription over time as new products become available and personal preferences change. This avoids both taste fatigue and boredom (Blow *et al.*, 2005) and the risk of poor adherence to their diet. Many manufacturers will offer product samples to try prior to ordering them on regular prescription and individuals need information from relevant healthcare professionals concerning these sources, particularly as many of the products are available only on prescription.

Those paying for their prescriptions should also be reminded of the cost savings by applying for a certificate of prepayment of prescription charges (FP95).

The third shopping list is the most difficult and requires the most vigilance and this is the list of processed foods. Basically, these are those foods which have gone through a manufacturing process and either contain gluten or are at risk of containing gluten from cross-contamination. As we have already seen, labelling laws are complex and it takes some time to become accustomed to interpreting them. There is a wealth of information available from coeliac organizations (i.e. Coeliac U.K.) regarding safe shopping, and many publish food and drink directories or lists of those products safe to eat and these are especially useful, if not vital, until patients become more comfortable with their diet. Most supermarkets have a 'free from' aisle with specialist products for those with particular dietary needs. Many of these products will be expensive and include those staple items, like bread, available on prescription.

Table 5.3　Minimum monthly gluten free food prescription requirements for adults with coeliac disease

Age group	Suggested number of units per month	Example of minimum monthly prescription	
Male (19–59 years)	18	10 × 400 g loaves of bread (or 5 × 500 g mix suitable for making bread) 1 × (2 × 110/180 g) pizza bases	1 × 500 g pasta 2 × 200 g crackers/crisp breads 1 × 200 g sweet biscuits 1 × 500 g flour mix
Male (60–74 years)	16	10 × 400 g loaves of bread (or 5 × 500 g mix suitable for making bread) 1 × 500 g cake mix	1 × 500 g pasta 1 × 200 g crackers/crisp breads 1 × 200 g sweet biscuits
Male (75+ years)	14	8 × 400 g loaves of bread (or 4 × 500 g mix suitable for making bread) 1 × 500 g cake mix	1 × 500 g pasta 1 × 200 g crackers/crisp breads 1 × 200 g sweet biscuits
Female (19–74 years)	14	8 × 400 g loaves of bread (or 4 × 500 g mix suitable for making bread) 1 × (2 × 110/180 g) pizza bases	1 × 500 g pasta 2 × 200 g crackers/crisp breads 1 × 200 g sweet biscuits
Female (75+ years)	12	6 × 400 g loaves of bread (or 3 × 500 g mix suitable for making bread) 1 × 500 g cake mix	1 × 500 g pasta 1 × 200 g crackers/crisp breads 1 × 200 g sweet biscuits
Breastfeeding	Add four units	1 × 400 g loaf of bread	1 × 500 g pasta 1 × 200 g crackers/crisp breads
Third trimester of pregnancy	Add one unit		1 × 200 g sweet biscuits
High physical activity level	Add four units		1 × 500 g pasta 1 × 200 g crackers/crisp breads 1 × 200 g sweet biscuits

Blow *et al.* (2005), p. 12.

With experience coeliac shoppers will be able to identify the cheaper alternatives. By joining National Coeliac Organizations, patients will benefit from food directories, and by joining local affiliated or independent coeliac groups as well, they will also benefit from networking with others with coeliac disease in their area and be able to identify those local independent retailers providing gluten free items from local sources. In addition, government organizations like the Food Standards Agency (FSA) allow people to subscribe to automatic email alerts when products are withdrawn from sale, either because of incorrect or missing labelling or because of cross-contamination. The principles of these shopping lists are once again summarised in Table 5.4.

Cooking without gluten

If an individual was not keen on cooking before they were diagnosed with coeliac disease that position is unlikely to change on diagnosis, although many will invest in a bread maker, finding ready-made gluten free breads an acquired taste! For those who dislike cooking they are likely to have more difficulty in finding alternatives to ready meals, which are almost always gluten laden. This group includes in particular individuals living alone, especially the elderly. Very often these people will require the greatest dietetic input and support. For those who regularly cook from scratch, whether from love or necessity, cross-contamination will be a significant issue in the handling and preparation of food. The symptoms at diagnosis and the degree of mucosal damage and malabsorption will determine an individual's sensitivity to even low levels of gluten and the precautions that need to be taken. Additional advice that should be given to patients especially those with apparent resistant disease will be dealt with further on.

Medications

Many medications whether prescribed or purchased over the counter will contain gluten. The labelling requirements for

Table 5.4 Summary of shopping lists for coeliac diets

Shopping list	Items on list	Additional comments
One (weekly)	Foods that are gluten free in their natural state. Fruit, vegetables, meats, milk and eggs.	Take care where meats have been packaged that they have not been seasoned or contain stuffing.
Two (monthly)	Prescription foods. Gluten free prescribable items allocated a 'unit' value based on their carbohydrate and energy content and their cost.	Write a list of foods consumed prior to onset of symptoms to workout 'units' required per month. Access manufacturers for free samples of gluten free products. Do not overstock. Those paying for prescriptions should consider purchasing a pre-payment certificate (FP95).
Three	Foods which have gone through a manufacturing process and either contain gluten or are at risk of containing gluten from cross-contamination.	Use coeliac organization's food & drink directories to identify safe and unsafe foods. Local coeliac groups share information regarding local sources of gluten free products. The Food Standards Agency has an automatic email alert service for when gluten free products are withdrawn from sale. Specialist gluten free products are often more expensive and many are available on prescription.

medications in relation to gluten are identical to those applied to pre-packed foods (Shepherd & Gibson, 2006). All medications should therefore be checked for gluten. Obviously, where there are no alternatives, gluten-containing medications may have to be taken where the overall risk to health from not taking them is greater. Advice regarding medication use should always be sought from an appropriately trained healthcare professional.

Activity

Is there a procedure in place for medication reviews when individuals with coeliac disease are admitted to hospital?

Eating out

This is the arena where all coeliac patients potentially feel unsafe and uncomfortable. One health economics research project (Coeliac U.K., 2007) showed that 67% of coeliac patients are unlikely to eat a meal outside of their home. Having become 'expert' in reading and interpreting food labels and storing, preparing and cooking gluten free foods, they are aware of the difficulty in maintaining a gluten free environment and are all the more suspicious of establishments that cater for both those on a gluten-containing and gluten free diet. Cross-contamination is perhaps the biggest issue and so knowledge of the possible sources as highlighted in Figure 5.1 will allow individuals to question what they are eating when away from home. Once again local coeliac groups will provide an invaluable source of information on establishments (cafes, public houses, restaurants, hotels) catering for those on a gluten free diet and specialist clinics can be an additional source of information by collecting patients' personal recommendations.

As with processed food there can be a lot of hidden gluten in foods when eating out. For example, a baked potato with cheese would seem a safe gluten free lunch to pick from a menu, but what if the cheese was packed pre-grated? There is a risk that flour has been used to keep the cheese gratings separate. Telephoning ahead to check whether establishments cater for a gluten free diet might be a nuisance but provides a measure of reassurance and hassle-free dining. Patients should not be afraid to challenge, not only what foods are provided but how they are prepared and cooked. Obviously, this is more difficult when attending private functions such as birthday parties; many people with severe allergies get around this by preparing and taking their own food.

For those with coeliac disease even greater difficulty is encountered when planning holidays and many coeliac patients return year on year to the same resort/destination/hotel using the same travel companies in the safe knowledge that their dietary needs are catered for. The very purpose of a holiday is to feel relaxed and the potential stress of an uncertain environment can put off all but the very confident traveller or poorly compliant coeliac; surveys (Zarkadas, 2006) have shown that 38% avoid travel altogether, but with careful planning and the help from national coeliac organizations many airlines, travel companies and resorts now cater ably for those requiring special diets.

Hospital admissions are another area of difficulty for coeliac patients. Surprisingly, many nurses fail to recognise or act on the need for a gluten free diet in the hospital setting. This situation is common with many special diets that fall outside of supposedly normal nutritional requirements but given the increasing prevalence should be more easily catered for. As with eating in a restaurant, patients will need to feel confident regarding issues of food preparation and cross-contamination. The dietitian should be alerted as soon as a patient with coeliac disease is admitted, so that the appropriate foods can be arranged and reassurance provided.

Activity

Find out from your catering department what the dietary provision for coeliac patients is in your clinical area, especially bread. Is it satisfactory?

The role of the healthcare professional

Even in researching and writing this chapter, I have come to admire all those individuals with any food allergy including coeliac disease, who have to maintain a constant vigilance over what they eat. I often challenge students to pretend that they have coeliac disease for a day and to keep a record of their dietary intake for that day and identify the food items eaten that contained gluten. A similar exercise is to write out their usual shopping list and then to look for gluten free alternatives on their next visit to the supermarket. I personally never get past the 'free from' aisle.

The key principles for establishing a gluten free diet as the treatment for coeliac disease are as follows:

- Initial dietetic input to assess individual nutritional needs and education as to which foods contain gluten, which foods are safe to eat and how to maintain a balanced diet.
- Acknowledgement that coeliac disease is a life-long diagnosis and not something you grow out of.
- If in doubt – leave it out. Then seek advice from national or local support groups or healthcare professionals on the products suitability.
- Encouragement to join national and local coeliac organizations.
- Education on food labelling and interpreting food labels including Codex safety standards.
- Making three shopping lists and confidently accessing the items on each of them.
- Being aware of the potential sources of cross-contamination with gluten.
- Being confident in challenging food manufacturers and caterers concerning both the source and the preparation of food and food ingredients.

Healthcare professionals need to remember that establishing a life-long adherence to a gluten free diet takes time and necessitates making a few mistakes along the way. In addition to dietetic advice and support, nurses in a variety of settings will meet and care for individuals with coeliac disease. With a good working knowledge of the disease they can provide ongoing support and education, either directly or by referral to the appropriate agency.

HINTS AND TIPS

- Meet with the dietitians to discuss how your roles will compliment each other. Explore the opportunity to have occasional joint clinics where new coeliac patients can see both the dietitian and the nurse specialist at the same visit.
- Look at the provision of gluten free foods for inpatients with coeliac disease. Work together with the caterers and dietitians to improve the foods available.
- Think about how you will provide support for these patients in the early stages after diagnosis? A number of suggestions are:
  - Helpline
  - 'Frequently asked questions' information sheets
  - Local and national coeliac groups
  - Focus groups
  - Websites
  - Buddy up with other coeliac patients of similar age/background.
- Ask patients to recommend local places to eat, restaurants, cafes, pubs etc. that cater for coeliac disease and put together a local list which you can give to new patients. Remember to update it regularly!
- Make a collection of 'gluten free' recipes as they appear in magazines to give out as copies to new patients.

REFERENCES

Blow, C., Butt, S., Buxton, A., Holmes, G., Jenkins, H., Lowdon, J., McGough, N. & Wylie, C. (2005) *Gluten Free Foods: A Prescribing Guide.* Good Relations Healthcare, London. http://www.glutenfreefood.co.uk/Gluten free%20foods% 20-%20Prescribing%20Guidelines%202005.pdf. Accessed 18 June 2007.

Canadian Food Inspection Agency (2003) Gluten free foods definition. In *Guide to Food Labelling and Advertising.*

Point 9.9.4, Section B24.018. http://www.inspection.gc.ca/english/fssa/labeti/guide/ch9ae.shtml. Accessed 1 June 2007.

Case, S. (2005) The Gluten free diet: How to provide effective education and resources. *Gastroenterology* 128:S128–S134.

Catassi, C., Fabiani, E., Iacono, G., D'Agate, C., Francaville, R., Biagi, F., Volta, U., Aecomando, S., Picarelli, A., DeVitis, I., Picanelli, G., Gesuita, R., Carle, F., Madolesi, A., Bearzi, I. & Fasano, A. (2007) A prospective double-blind placebo-controlled trial to establish a safe gluten threshold for patients with coeliac disease. *American Journal of Clinical Nutrition* 85(1):160–166.

Coeliac Sprue Association. *Use of the Term 'Gluten Free'.* http://www.csaceliacs.org/DefofGlutenFree.php. Accessed 1 June 2007.

Codex Alimentarius Commission (1981) *Codex Standard for 'Gluten free Foods' Codex Standard 118-1981 (Amended 1983).* http://www.codexalimentarius.net/download/standards/291/cxs_118e.pdf. Accessed 31 May 2007.

Coeliac U.K. (2007) Health economics research project. *Crossed Grain* 68:35.

Coeliac U.K. (2008) *New Codex Standard.* http://www.coeliac.org.uk/healthcare_professionals/healthcare_newsletter/895.asp?dm_i=205935322. Accessed 16 July 2008.

Collin, P., Thorell, L., Kaukinen, K. & Maki, M. (2004) The safe threshold for gluten contamination in gluten free products. Can trace amounts be accepted in the treatment of coeliac disease? *Alimentary Pharmacology and Therapeutics* 19:1277–1283.

Danowski, L., Brand, L.G. & Connolly, J. (2003) Selections from current literature: Gluten free diets, coeliac disease and associated disorders. *Family Practice* 20(5):607–611.

European Union Labelling Directive (2003) Directive of 2003/89/3c of the European parliament and of the council of 10th November 2003 amending directive 2000/13/EC as regards indication of the ingredients present in foodstuffs. *Official Journal of the European Union* L308:15–18.

Fasano A. & Cattasi, C. (2001) Current approaches to the diagnosis and treatment of coeliac disease: An evolving spectrum. *Gastroenterology* 120(3):636–651.

Food Standards Agency (2006) *Guidance on Allergen Management and Consumer Information.* FSA/1064/0606. http://www.food.gov.uk/multimedia/pdfs/maycontainguide.pdf. Accessed 5 June 2007.

Her Majesty's Stationery Office (1987) *Statutory Instrument No 1680 (C51). The Consumer Protection Act* (Commencement No, 1). HMSO, London.

Her Majesty's Stationery Office (1996) *Statutory Instrument No. 1499. The Food Labelling Regulations as Amended by the Food Labelling (Amendment) Regulations 1998 and The Food Labelling (Amendment) (No. 2) Regulation 1999.* HMSO, London.

Kupper, C. (2005) Dietary guidelines and implementation for coeliac disease. *Gastroenterology* 128:S121–S127.

Lee, A. (2005) Coeliac disease: Detection and treatment. *Topical Clinical Nutrition* 20:139–145.

Mills, E.N.C., Valovirta, E., Madsen, C., Taylor, S.L., Vieths, S., Anklam, E., Baumgartner, S., Koch, P., Crevel, R.L.W. & Frewer, L. (2004) Information provision for allergic consumers – where are we going with food allergen labelling? *Allergy* 99:1262–1268.

Shepherd, S. & Gibson, P.R. (2006) Understanding the gluten free diet for teaching in Australia. *Nutrition and Dietetics* 63:155–165.

Thompson, T., Dennis, M., Higgins, L.A., Lee, A.R. & Sharrett, M.K. (2005) Gluten free diet survey: Are Americans with coeliac disease consuming recommended amounts of fibre, iron, calcium and grain foods? *Journal of Human Nutritional Dietetics* 18:163–169.

Valdes, I., Garcia, E., Llorente, M. & Mendez, E. (2003) Innovative approach to low-level gluten determination in foods using a novel sandwich-linked immunosorbent assay protocol. *European Journal of Gastroenterology and Hepatology* 15:465–474.

Zarkadas, M., Cranney, A., Case, S., Molloy, M., Switzer, C., Graham, I.D., Butzner, J.D., Rashid, M., Warren, R.E. & Burrows, V. (2006) The impact of a gluten free diet on adults with coeliac disease: Results of a national survey. *Journal of Human Nutritional Dietetics* 19:41–49.

Chapter 6
Long-Term Support and Follow-Up

LEARNING OUTCOMES

At the end of this chapter you should be able to:

- Discuss the principles behind long-term follow-up care.
- Discuss the different methods of follow-up and the strengths and weaknesses of each.
- Describe what we are looking for at follow-up.
- List the key complications associated with coeliac disease and how these are managed.
- Describe the concept of the expert patient and their 'creation'.

Having acknowledged in the previous chapter that coming to terms with a gluten free diet takes time, long-term support and follow-up is a key consideration. Lapses in dietary compliance are not unusual even when patients have received expert education and advice. The restrictive nature of the diet, taste fatigue and peer pressure all contribute to lapses whether temporary or long term. It is easy to succumb to the odd biscuit or cake when popping to a friend's house for coffee, rather than appear rude or have to discuss your medical condition. It is easy to succumb to the occasional takeaway at the end of a busy day when you are too tired to cook. It is easy to sacrifice the gluten free diet when faced with other life-challenging events such as bereavement or divorce. The list of reasons is endless; anyone who has been on a weight-reducing diet will know just how attractive forbidden foods can be for all the same sorts of reasons. This alone should help us to understand the needs of this patient group. However, evidence unfortunately shows us that poor dietary compliance over a prolonged period can and does lead to potentially life-threatening complications.

The aim of this chapter is to emphasise the importance of the initial baseline assessment at diagnosis, to exclude associated concomitant conditions and to identify deficiencies in micronutrients, providing a benchmark against which to measure any future symptoms. We then look at how life-long dietary compliance is maintained with follow-up based on patient's needs, an undertaking that requires not only ongoing professional support but also peer group support to help create the expert patient. This chapter is the appropriate place to discuss again some of the complications of the disease as it highlights the importance of dietary compliance, which in turn highlights the need for long-term support and follow-up.

ASSESSMENT OF DIETARY COMPLIANCE

Successful management of coeliac disease requires a team approach, involving the person with coeliac disease, the family, the dietitian, the doctors and reputable coeliac support groups. Following on from the initial dietetic assessment, a medical review is essential to establish a baseline that will help determine the frequency and intensity of future follow-up. This is in addition to any continued support felt appropriate by the dietitians. This assessment can be done by appropriately trained nurses as part of an ongoing package of support, working within protocols or algorithms (Figure 6.1).

The baseline assessment is advisable at around 3 months after diagnosis, giving time for the initial dietetic review and enabling an initial appraisal of the response to treatment, which in 70% of adults will occur within weeks or days (BSG, 2002). The baseline and subsequent follow-ups will be very similar.

As discussed in Chapter 4, how the interview is conducted is crucial in establishing both trust and rapport. The principles

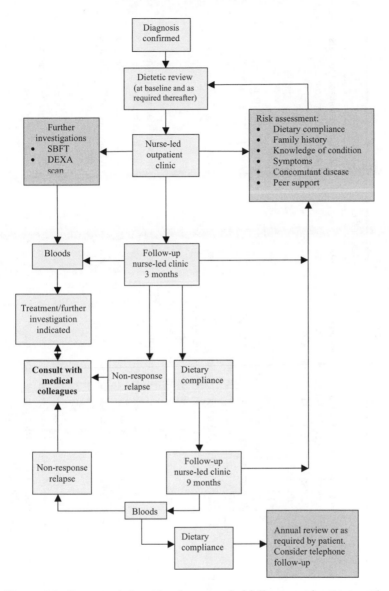

Figure 6.1   Suggested algorithm for nurse-led follow-up of patients with coeliac disease.

of follow-up and the rationale behind the questions asked and investigations ordered are outlined in Table 6.1; these will vary according to local protocols but should incorporate a sound up-to-date evidence base. The purpose of regular review in

Table 6.1 Principles and rationale behind baseline assessment and long-term follow-up

Questions to be addressed	Rationale	At baseline	At follow-up
Has the patient seen a dietitian?	Imperative at baseline to assess not only understanding of gluten free diet but to assess for other food intolerances and nutritional deficiencies.	Yes	Not unless patient requests or dietitian/clinician feel necessary
Does the patient need to be assessed at home?	Home dietetic review especially can be useful. In older patients cooking equipment, preparation areas and food storage can all hinder dietary compliance in the long term.	Yes	No Unless change in circumstances suggested
How does the patient feel?	Gives early indication of long-term compliance – if a patient feels worse on the diet less likely to be motivated to continue. Other symptoms may need investigation.	Yes	Yes
Does the patient understand why the gluten free diet is important?	Indicates level of education and whether further targeted education needed. Also assesses motivation.	Yes	If there is an indication of poor dietary compliance
Does the patient understand the association between their symptoms and coeliac disease?	Indicates level of education and also motivation.	Yes	If there is an indication of poor dietary compliance
History of concomitant disease (with particular attention to associated clinical disorders as outlined in Box 3.1 in Chapter 3)	May increase risk factors associated with poor dietary compliance, or may require closer follow-up and support and/or further investigation.	Yes	Yes Question any further illness since last review

(continued)

When was the last time you ate anything that you thought might contain gluten?	The single most useful question you can ask to assess dietary compliance. Cannot be answered with a 'yes' or 'no'.	Yes	Yes
Is the patient a member of any local/national coeliac organization?	Indicates ongoing motivation and education.	Yes	Yes
Quality-of-life issues – Is the diet affecting their day-to-day life?	These can be early indicators of a risk of dietary lapse. Look for indications of stress, work/life balance, relationship problems etc.	Yes	Yes
Is their weight stable?	With improved absorption some find that they put on additional weight and need help and support to overcome concerns. Persistent low weight or weight loss requires close monitoring and/or further evaluation.	Yes	Yes
Bone or joint pain.	Assesses known bone abnormality or new symptoms.	Yes	Yes
Any skin rashes?	Assesses for dermatitis herpetiformis.	Yes	Yes
Any change in bowel habit?	Indicates dietary compliance/resistant disease in those with symptoms pre diagnosis that included diarrhoea. Ongoing or new diagnosis of change in bowel habit will need further evaluation to exclude malignant pathology.	Yes	Yes

Table 6.1 *(continued)*

Questions to be addressed	Rationale	At baseline	At follow-up
Medication review. Prescribed non-prescribed and herbal medications.	Interaction with prescribed and self-administered medications may account for symptoms. In addition medications may contain gluten.	Yes	Yes

Investigations/tests to be considered	Rationale	At baseline	At follow-up
Bone densitometry (DEXA), following risk assessment.	To allow early treatment of any bone abnormality.	Yes	Individual follow-up as recommended at baseline
Small bowel follow through.	This is contentious; however, there is some merit given a risk of small bowel lymphoma up to 40 times greater that the general population. Capsule endoscopy may eventually replace as the investigation of choice.	Yes, dependent on local policy	No Unless symptoms indicate (i.e. lethargy, diarrhoea, weight loss)
Blood tests. FBC, iron studies including ferritin, folate, vitamin B12, vitamins A, D and E. Bone profile, LFTs U&Es, EMA.	To monitor compliance and complication risk.	Yes	Yes Not all will be necessary
Barium enema. Consider particularly in patients >45 years with persistent diarrhoea.	To exclude large bowel pathology.	No	If symptoms indicate

FBC, full blood count; LFTs, liver function tests; U&Es, urea and electrolytes; EMA, endomysial antibodies.

addition to checking compliance with and response to the gluten free diet also looks for evidence of decreased motivation, gaps in education and signs and symptoms indicating possible complications.

Activity

What are the principles behind follow-up within your clinical area? Are all patients followed up routinely and if so how?

Where possible close family especially a spouse, or parent in the case of young adults, should be encouraged to attend these early appointments, as they are the best-placed individuals to offer the long-term support and motivation and also as studies have shown (Sverker *et al.*, 2007) they can be equally affected by the disease, describing anxiety in social situations and also fear that they themselves will harm the individual with coeliac disease as a result of a mistake when cooking.

Follow-up will initially be at fairly regular intervals whilst the individual comes to terms with the changes in both diet and lifestyle. When the endomysial antibodies are normal and there are no clinical symptoms, then there is evidence that the patient is doing well and follow-up can be less frequent, based on individual needs. Annual review is still recommended (BSG, 2002; Pietzak, 2005), and this could be undertaken as a telephone consultation.

Telephone consultation

The telephone has been used as a tool for delivering health care since its invention in 1876. In fact, Alexander Graham Bell's first recorded telephone call was reputedly one for medical help after he spilt sulphuric acid on himself (Car & Sheikh, 2003). The public it would appear value the option of consulting over the telephone, citing benefits such as not sitting around for hours in waiting rooms and not having to travel or incur the cost to health and temper trying to park. A well-controlled coeliac patient may also question the time and cost, to walk into a consulting room simply to say *yes thank you I'm fine*, especially to find that 2 weeks down the line they experience problems and need then to re-negotiate medical review.

Nurses in specialist practice have used telephone advice lines for some time as a valuable contribution to care focused on promoting self-management strategies for individuals with long-term conditions (RCN, 2006), including those with coeliac disease. However, using the telephone to undertake a more formal consultation requires an additional range of skills. There is a need to be able to compensate for the inability to physically assess or examine the patient, requiring a more refined appreciation of the importance of verbal cues and focused history (Car *et al.*, 2004). What is the patient telling me; what are they not telling me?

Activity

The next time you receive a telephone call from a patient or relative, think about the verbal cues. Can you tell whether the person is anxious, angry etc. from the tone, speed, pitch and content of the language? Similarly, what verbal cues do you display when answering the call?

Telephone consultation does not suit everyone and patients should not only be given an option but be assessed as to their ability to use the telephone as a means of communication, if they actually have a telephone, which an estimated 10% of the population do not (Car *et al.*, 2004). Many older adults start to experience increasing difficulty in using their telephone, hearing problems, dexterity in using key pads, mobility in getting to the telephone in the first place are all issues that need to be considered. For some a visit to the hospital each year decreases the sense of isolation and loneliness felt in having the disease; it is surprising how much networking goes on in a hospital waiting room and patients should always have the option of a face-to-face consultation.

In setting up a telephone follow-up clinic, it is necessary to ensure that you have identified accurately the needs of the population at whom the service is aimed, that it is set up with a

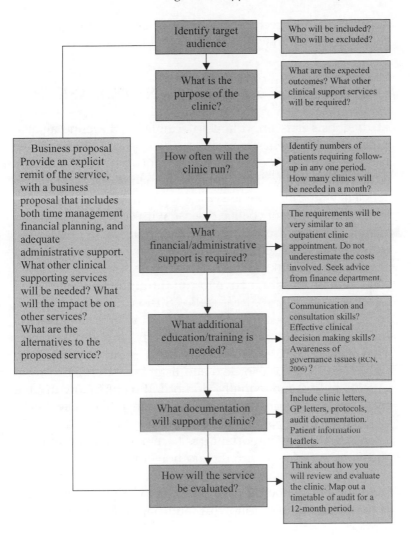

Figure 6.2 Setting up a telephone clinic.

clear business plan that includes financial and administrative support and that there are clear protocols guiding the content of the consultation and the documentation (RCN, 2006) (Figure 6.2).

Where antibodies remain elevated and clinical symptoms and nutritional deficiencies persist, these should prompt more frequent evaluation and closer monitoring to exclude other diagnoses and correct associated disorders; in these cases telephone consultation would not be suitable.

EXCLUSION OF CONCOMITANT DISEASE

At diagnosis it is important to establish a baseline against which all subsequent symptoms can be assessed. Here we have a chicken-and-egg scenario, as some concomitant disease may actually have led to the diagnosis of coeliac disease, i.e. iron deficiency anaemia. Some symptoms may take a time to unravel; a diagnosis of coeliac disease with so many associated clinical disorders (see section 'Risk of Malignancy Associated with Coeliac Disease') can become the panacea for all ills, and it is important to take each symptom on its own merit. It is neither prudent nor productive to run through the whole list of possible concomitant diseases (Box 3.1 in Chapter 3) with every newly diagnosed patient, unless we intend to increase the emotional isolation and fear they already commonly express (Sverker *et al.*, 2005). It is rather a case of being mindful of the possible associated disorders and listening carefully to what patients tell us and, equally, do not tell us at follow-up; the questions and suggested investigations in Table 6.1 will help identify the more common associated conditions. Case study 6.1 highlights how important it is to remain vigilant for complications associated with dietary non-compliance. Although already discussed in Chapter 3, the purpose of discussing the exclusion of osteoporosis again here is to heighten awareness of the importance of follow-up and ongoing education and support.

Case study 6.1

A 69-year-old gentleman, Mr P, who lives alone, was diagnosed with coeliac disease in 1999. Non-compliant with his diet, frequent face-to-face follow-up was needed at which he admitted to eating normal bread, beer and cake. Despite intensive education and support from both the nurses and the dietitians he persisted in consuming gluten. His DEXA scan confirmed osteoporosis, his endomysial antibodies remained positive and vitamin A, D and E levels were persistently low. Mr P's main reason for non-compliance was that he felt entirely well and was reluctant to give up foods that he loved, despite the evidence that it was causing damage in terms of nutrient deficiencies and malabsorption leading to osteoporosis. It was suspected that living alone may also have played a part as he was reliant on his own cooking skills and therefore often relied on convenience foods.

At each clinic visit he promised to make changes to his diet but no changes were forthcoming.

A breakthrough was finally made in 2006 where he suddenly converted to a gluten free diet, ordering his bread on prescription and exchanging his beer for whiskey! He had also joined Coeliac U.K. and was following their guidance on safe foods. He was able to provide us with an outline of his diet which suggested that he was actually making a genuine effort, although he was now eating only two meals a day. There was noted however to have been a 6-kg weight loss since his appointment 12 months earlier. There were no bowel symptoms and bloods although not normal were showing an improvement and therefore it was felt that the weight loss could be ascribed to the changes in his diet. It was decided to review him in a further 4 months and as with all patients he knew to contact the helpline should he experience any problems in the intervening period. At his next appointment it was felt that Mr P looked pale and there was noted to be further weight loss. He admitted to feeling tired but assured us that he was adhering to his diet and reported no change in bowel habit or other symptoms. Bloods showed iron deficiency anaemia, positive endomysial antibodies and low vitamin levels. A CT scan was therefore arranged and showed a colonic wall thickening just proximal to the hepatic flexure. Colonoscopy showed a colonic carcinoma at the hepatic flexure. Mr P underwent a right hemicolectomy and cholecystectomy as there was found to be tumour extending into the gall bladder. Histology showed a high-grade malignant T-cell non-Hodgkin's lymphoma and Mr P is now undergoing radiotherapy.

Osteoporosis

As discussed in Chapter 3, osteoporosis is now thought to be the most important long-term medical concern for those with coeliac disease (Walters, 2007). By the age of 30 peak bone mass is reached. Therefore, coeliac patients diagnosed before that age need to maintain calcium and exercise levels to ensure maximum bone density and better bone health later in life, whilst those diagnosed over the age of 30 and certainly post-menopausal or in the case of men over 55 may need calcium supplementation in addition to a calcium-rich diet and more moderate exercise.

Activity

Revise your knowledge on the growth and turnover of bone. Assess yourself against the risk factors associated with loss of bone density.

Although now no longer widely advocated (BSG, 2007), screening newly diagnosed coeliac patients for signs of reduced bone mineral density is useful to provide a baseline for education, treatment and support. There are a number of risk assessment tools available but no clear criteria as to how many factors constitute a 'risk', which is why the DEXA scan at diagnosis provides the foundation on which to base future education and monitoring. The key risks are:

- If female – early menopause (before 45 years), early hysterectomy (before 50 years), irregular or infrequent menstrual periods during life. These all result in early loss of oestrogen, the major hormone influencing bone growth. After the age of 30, both men and women start to lose bone density as a natural part of aging.
- Long-term use of high-dose corticosteroids (i.e. 7.5 mg daily or more for >6 months).
- Smoking – has a toxic effect on bone, preventing the construction of new bone.
- Alcohol intake – should be within the recommended units. Apart from damaging the skeleton, too much alcohol also increases the risk of falls.
- Immobility – weight-bearing exercise is the best way to increase bone strength and therefore those bed bound or elderly are at greater risk, immobility accounting for up to a 40% loss of bone density.

- Lack of sunshine – the main source of vitamin D is the sun through our skin, which the body then converts to vitamin D and stores in the fat. Vitamin D is essential in the absorption of calcium. Therefore, those who rarely go outside or who are well covered up on religious or cultural ground are at high risk.
- Low calcium intake – those avoiding dairy produce or who are on a reducing diet are obviously at risk.
- Other diseases – i.e. liver, thyroid, cushings.
- Family history of osteoporosis – importantly, around 80% of our bone health is inherited from our parents.
- Unexplained fractures – a history of unexplained fractures could indicate existing osteoporosis.
- Low weight for height (BMI < 20) – increases the fracture risk. Again reduces oestrogen levels in both men and women.

Having identified the relevant risk factors and assessed bone density this then allows targeted education strategies to improve bone health in addition to appropriate treatments for existing osteopenia/osteoporosis (see Table 6.2). The mainstay of education centres on getting enough calcium and vitamin D and regular exercise.

Exercise – is important not only in strengthening bone mass and preventing age-related loss but in increasing muscle strength and thereby supporting the joints and helping to prevent falls. However, any positive gain in bone strength is lost when exercising ceases, so any exercise should consist of sustainable regimes such as a 30-min brisk walk two to three times a week, rather than the good intentioned 5-km run that falters after 1 km and is never attempted again. Parking the car in the furthest corner of the car park rather than right outside of the door of the supermarket is a positive move or taking the stairs one or two floors instead of the lift. Obviously where osteoporosis is diagnosed the exercise regime should be adjusted accordingly, as some forms of exercise will simply not be manageable.

Calcium – almost all of the body's calcium comes from the diet, calcium that is essential for building and maintaining

Table 6.2 Treatment of osteopenia and osteoporosis

Osteopenia at any age	1. Strict adherence to a gluten free diet. 2. Encourage regular weight-bearing exercise. 3. Ensure adequate dietary calcium with calcium supplementation to ensure daily intake of 1000 mg a day. 4. Lifestyle advice, re-smoking, alcohol intake.
In post-menopausal women or men >55 years, if high number of risk factors or previous history of fragility fracture	1. Treat as for osteoporosis.
Osteoporosis in pre-menopausal women or men <55 years	1. As 1–4 above. 2. Due to lack of appropriate trials (BSG, 2007), bisphosphonates should be used with caution where there is indication of high risk or history of previous fragility fracture. Re-evaluate with DEXA after 2–3 years, discontinue treatment if adequate response and treat as osteopenia.
Osteoporosis in post-menopausal women or men >55 years	1. As 1–4 above. 2. Long-term oral bisphosphonate. If intolerant consider (from BSG, 2007): Raloxifene – An oestrogen receptor modulator. Useful for use in post-menopausal women unlike HRT does not increase risk of coronary heart disease and decreases risk of invasive breast cancer. Teriparatide – A human recombinant parathyroid hormone. Given by daily subcutaneous injection. Licensed for use for 18 months only. Calcitonin – A naturally occurring hormone inhibiting bone resorption by osteoclasts. Taken weekly by intranasal spray.
All men with osteoporosis	1. In addition to recommendations as above consider hypogonadism and check blood testosterone levels *after* treatment with a gluten free diet and replace if low, using daily skin patches (BSG, 2007). *Prior to a gluten free diet androgen resistance will cause high testosterone levels.*

HRT, hormone replacement therapy.

Table 6.3 Examples of sources of calcium

Source of calcium	Quantity	Typical value (mg)
Lean rump steak	100 g	5
Apple	Medium	7
Roast chicken (skin off)	100 mg	16
Strawberries	150 g	19
Orange	Medium	35
Dried apricots	50 g	35
Almonds	50 g	110
Tinned salmon (with bones)	100 g	220
Full fat milk	250 mL	285
Skimmed milk	250 mL	320
Tinned sardines (with bones)	100 g	380
Plain yoghurt	200 g	390

bone strength. Intake of calcium and its absorption is important. Absorption is reduced by excessive alcohol and caffeine,
soft drinks containing phosphates (i.e. carbonated drinks) and
foods high in animal proteins. Calcium is also lost through the
skin, nails, sweat and urine, the latter an increased risk in diets
high in salt.

For adults the recommended daily intake of calcium is
1000 mg a day. This rises to 1300 mg a day in teenagers, young
pregnant mothers, menopausal women and men over the age
of around 70.

Calcium is found in varying quantities in a number of food
groups, with the smallest quantities found in meat and fresh
fruit (see Table 6.3). The highest source of calcium is found
in dairy products, and contrary to expectations the lower the
fat content the higher the calcium content, so skimmed milk
has a higher calcium content than full-cream milk. This can
be an issue for coeliac patients with a lactose intolerance and
therefore an intolerance to many dairy products. This is where
dietetic input is essential.

Hyposplenism

Hyposplenism occurs where the spleen functions poorly and
although I have stated that there are disorders that should
be excluded it is difficult to determine the incidence of

hyposplenism. However, it is worth mentioning here as patients with coeliac disease often question their need for vaccination against pneumococcal infection, an infection associated with coeliac disease and thought by some (Wright, 1995) to be a major complication of the disease.

Pneumococcus is a gram-positive bacteria recognised as a major cause of pneumonia in the late nineteenth century. Despite the name, the organism causes many types of infection other than pneumonia, including acute sinusitis, otitis media, meningitis, osteomyelitis, septic arthritis, endocarditis, peritonitis, pericarditis, cellulitis and brain abscess.

There is, as already stated, difficulty in determining the incidence in coeliac disease, which varies from a third (Corazza *et al.*, 1999) to three-quarters of all adult patients (O'Grady *et al.*, 1984). In these particular studies the large discrepancy is thought to be explained by genetic heterogeneity between the Irish and Italian population.

Although the cause is unknown, speculation postulates the absorption of antigens through damaged small bowel mucosa and the formation of antigen/antibody complexes (Wright, 1995). The haematological manifestations that assess splenic function are complex but briefly include the presence of pitting red blood cells (PRC) and Howell–Jolly bodies, which are histopathological findings of basophilic nuclear remnants (clusters of DNA) in young erythrocytes during the response to severe haemolytic anaemia, megaloblastic anaemia, splenectomy, or due to a damaged spleen, present in conditions such as hyposplenism. Corazza *et al.* (1999) also showed low Tuftsin activity in coeliac patients, even when the PRC percentage was within normal range. Tuftsin is a naturally occurring peptide relating to the immune system function and deficiency results in increased susceptibility to certain infections. Tuftsin and PRC measurements are the most sensitive and easily replicable tests of splenic function but are not routinely used at present to assess splenic function in coeliac patients.

Despite the apparent risk of hyposplenism there is little published evidence of mortality resulting from infection (Johnston & Robinson, 1998) and even then there are questions arising (Parnell *et al.*, 1998) as to the certainty of the diagnosis where complex concomitant medical problems exist. So, what are the risks to patients with coeliac disease?

The severity of hyposplenism appears to increase with age at diagnosis and duration of exposure to gluten (Corazza *et al.*, 1999; McKay *et al.*, 1993; Muller & Toghill, 1995; Wright, 1995), the main factor being pre-exposure to gluten. Some early studies (O'Grady *et al.*, 1984) show improvement in splenic dysfunction after removal of gluten from the diet. Splenic atrophy or asplenia, referring to the absence of normal splenic function, is far less well defined in coeliac disease and has a mixed response to the removal of gluten.

There is evidence (Mckinley *et al.*, 1995) of an appropriate antibody response to pneumococcal antigens in both splenic dysfunction and splenic atrophy, with suggestions that in view of the potential fluctuation in immunologic integrity in coeliac disease, vaccination should be considered for all patients. This is supported in theory in the publication *Immunisation against infection diseases* (HMSO, 1996) that recommends pneumococcal vaccine for:

> Asplenia or severe dysfunction of the spleen, including homozygous sickle cell disease and coeliac syndrome (p. 168).

The suggestion here however is that vaccination is only given with evidence of splenic dysfunction rather than simply because the individual has coeliac disease.

Given the increasing number of patients with coeliac disease, the small numbers of reported fatalities associated with pneumococcal infection and the difficulty in determining the incidence of hyposplenism, blanket vaccination and revaccination are not really feasible. However, patients should be given appropriate information and advice about hyposplenism as a possible complication of coeliac disease and its association with poor dietary compliance, with the recommendation that:

- To minimise the risk of severe infection if splenic function is impaired, patients should seek medical advice in case of fever and consider annual flu vaccination.
- Given the increased risk of hyposplenism with long pre-exposure to gluten, patients with a late diagnosis of coeliac disease should consider the risks and benefits of

pneumococcal vaccination and discuss this with a medical practitioner.

Activity

Look up the drug profiles of both the flu and pneumococcal vaccines.

RISK OF MALIGNANCY ASSOCIATED WITH COELIAC DISEASE

It is accepted by most that there is an increased risk of malignancy associated with coeliac disease. With an increased risk of non-Hodgkin's lymphoma, oesophageal cancer and small bowel lymphoma in particular reported in a variety of studies. The association was first described in the early 1960s (Gough *et al.*, 1962) but what is the magnitude of that risk? This question is particularly relevant in the long-term follow-up of patients, many of whom will question the level of risk and its association with dietary compliance.

The best known data regarding malignancy in coeliac disease come from a series of studies in the United Kingdom in Derby (Holmes *et al.*, 1989) that looked at a cohort of patients with coeliac disease over a period of 19 years and found that in patients who had been on a gluten free diet for more than 5 years the risk of malignancy was no higher than that in the general population but that in those not adhering to the diet the risk of malignancy was increased. How dietary compliance was assessed is unclear but the fact that there has been an interest in coeliac disease in Derby for many years may mean that follow-up assessment and monitoring of their dietary compliance is more thorough than anywhere else, resulting in a lower risk of malignancy than in a more symptomatic population. A possibility identified by the authors themselves in a more recent publication (Card *et al.*, 2004) actually calculated a lower risk of small bowel lymphoma than previously thought, which may also have to do with our increased recognition of the disease in asymptomatic patients. Few studies have explored the differences between symptomatic and asymptomatic patients (Goddard & Gillett, 2006).

Some studies found that the modest increase in the relative and absolute risk of malignancy and mortality in people with coeliac disease occurred between 1 and 3 years after diagnosis (Corrao *et al.*, 2001; West *et al.*, 2004) and slowly decreased between 3 and 5 years (Card *et al.*, 2004; Holmes *et al.*, 1989). It is difficult to say with certainty that those early malignancies were as a result of coeliac disease and of course possible that a proportion of them had a malignancy that precipitated the diagnosis of coeliac disease or had a low-grade lymphoma and not coeliac disease at all, having a similar histological appearance (Goddard & Gillett, 2006). However, if the risk appears to decrease over time there must be some link to the protective effect of adhering to a gluten free diet. The fact that coeliac disease may arise in individuals who have been treated with a gluten free diet for some years would appear to contradict the beneficial effects of dietary compliance. However, as pointed out by Catassi *et al.* (2005) it is probably dependent on the total exposure time to dietary gluten in affected people rather than the time from diagnosis. Therefore, a relatively short time on a gluten free diet may be inadequate to turn round the effects of exposure to an oncologenic stimulant that may have been present for many years. This again links to changes from the previous classic disease presentation to those with atypical symptoms and the early identification of those affected individuals.

Similarly, the effects of continued ingestion of small amounts of gluten and cancer development have never been fully studied (Catassi *et al.*, 2005), remembering previous discussion regarding Codex standards and the difficulty in completely avoiding any dietary gluten.

It would appear that the majority of people with coeliac disease are now over the age of 40 when diagnosed (Card *et al.*, 2004) and small intestinal cancer itself is a disease of older people, with 90% affected over the age of 40 (Shack *et al.*, 2006). Although small intestinal cancer remains an uncommon malignancy its incidence has been increasing since the 1980s (Shack *et al.*, 2006). With an aging population and increasing numbers of asymptomatic patients being screened and diagnosed with coeliac disease, there is the possibility that there will be an increasing trend. With a five times greater incidence of non-Hodgkin's lymphoma and a 40 times greater incidence of small bowel lymphoma amongst coeliac patients than in the general population, no matter how small the risk, strict adherence to a gluten free diet appears to be the only possibility of preventing these rare but aggressive forms of cancer in this patient group. Case study 6.1 highlights one particular case of non-Hodgkin's lymphoma diagnosed 8 years after the diagnosis of coeliac disease.

Activity

Read Case study 6.1. Look up the signs, symptoms, diagnosis, treatment and management of non-Hodgkin's lymphoma. Think about how you might support a coeliac patient with this suspected malignancy. What might be the particular psychological issues for this patient thinking about the association with coeliac disease and more specifically timing of diagnosis, investigations, compliance with diet and symptoms?

SUPPORT GROUPS – THE EXPERT PATIENT

Good health is taken for granted by those of us lucky enough to have it and arises as an issue only when something upsets the balance and makes us 'ill'. Even then if we can control our symptoms we learn to frame that illness according to how it affects our everyday lives. Therefore, it stands to reason that if people become more involved in managing their health, they become better able to deal with long-standing or chronic illness including coeliac disease.

The British Government sets out its plans to create an expert patient's programme designed to encourage people to take responsibility for their health (Department of Health, 1999, 2001), followed on by an intention to make it easier for people to choose healthy lives by making available better information, tackling inequality issues and health promotion (Department of Health, 2004).

Activity

Are expert patient programmes available within your area? Find out how they are accessed and what they involve.

The doctor–patient relationship has changed from the paternalistic model of 'doctor knows best', with patients as mere recipients of care, to a partnership approach. Patients may actually be more risk averse than their doctors think, and so instead of underplaying patients' desire for information and participation, if we allow them to play a more active role in decision based on evidence as to why adherence to a gluten free diet is beneficial then this may prove more effective in motivating long-term behaviour change. Simply telling a patient that by adhering to a gluten free diet their symptoms will improve will work only if they had symptoms in the first place (which often they do not) or until they find that by doing so they put on weight because they start to absorb nutrients or become social recluses because of the dietary restrictions. Patients then fall into the category of 'difficult' or 'non-compliant' leading to more constructive confrontation, reducing even further any likely behaviour change.

The initial key then to becoming an expert patient is information, knowledge that empowers patients to become more active participants in their care.

The sheer volume of health information available is daunting, especially with the advent of the internet. Moreover, the information available is not always reliable or accurate and so an important role for nurses undertaking follow-up is to source and make readily available good-quality, evidence-based information. Hand in hand with this goes the concept of health literacy (Toofany, 2007), described as the capacity to obtain, interpret, assimilate and utilise basic health information. The level of 'health literacy' will determine patients' ability to self-manage and be dependent on factors such as basic reading and writing skills and their ability to critically analyse information.

Being an expert patient is not a soft option. It means taking responsibility. It means knowing and understanding the risks and benefits of non-compliance with treatment. Voluntary coeliac organizations and patient groups provide enormous support to people with coeliac disease and their families and play an increasing and vital role in disseminating knowledge and personal involvement in improving health. Membership of both national and local groups should be strongly encouraged. National groups provide support but in addition campaign and fund research into the disease, always with the thought of finding a cure. They work to raise awareness of the disease and the need for speedy diagnosis and robust aftercare.

Local groups meanwhile provide much-needed peer support, local knowledge and access to local events dependent on the group dynamics. Our local coeliac group, for example, organises cookery demonstrations, food fairs, coffee mornings, Christmas lunches and a host of other activities in addition to regular meetings.

Activity

Find out if there is a local active coeliac group in your area?

What all these organizations do imperatively is shown sufferers that they are not alone and provide the level of support required by the individual. Nurses involved in the follow-up of patients can provide additional support by collecting recipes and asking other coeliac patients to recommend gluten free products, recipes and restaurants that can be shared with other patients.

The importance of long-term support and follow-up is to ensure that coeliac disease does not take over the lives of sufferers or appear to offer limited options rather than real choice. How successful patients are in tackling the diagnosis of coeliac disease successfully depends much on their motivation to commit to changing behaviour that will both improve their symptoms and limit the long-term risks associated with non-compliance as already discussed. Their intention at that point in time to comply with a gluten free diet will be determined by the initial support and education they receive at the point of diagnosis and an accurate assessment of their motivation and capability change in the longer term.

HINTS AND TIPS

- Map out how the nurse led follow-up service will look. Think about the frequency, the mode of follow-up and the investigations.
- With the appropriate evidence agree with your medical colleagues whether the baseline small bowel investigations, DEXA scans and pneumococcal/flu vaccinations will form part of your follow-up as standard. Think about who will make the referrals and the associated local policies if you intend to refer yourself.
- Think about your strategies for dealing with the non-compliant patient. Who will you involve? How will you handle the interview? Ask a colleague to sit in at a patient interview with you and give you constructive feedback.
- Link with other nurse providing specialist services for patients with coeliac disease.

REFERENCES

British Society of Gastroenterology (2002) *Guidelines for the Management of Patients with Coeliac Disease.* BSG, London.

British Society of Gastroenteorlogy (2007) *Guidelines for Osteoporosis in inflammatory Bowel Disease and Coeliac Disease.* BSG, London.

Car, J., Freeman, G.K., Partridge, M.R. & Sheikh, A. (2004) Improving the quality and safety of telephone based delivery of care: Teaching telephone consultation skills (Editorial). *British Medical Journal* 13:2–3.

Car, J. & Sheikh, A. (2003) Telephone consultations. *British Medical Journal* 326:966–969.

Card, T.R., West, J. & Holmes, G.K.T. (2004) Risk of malignancy in diagnosed coeliac disease: A 24 year prospective, population-based, cohort study. *Alimentary Pharmacology and Therapeutics* 20:769–775.

Catassi, C., Bearzi, I. & Holmes, K. (2005) Association of coeliac disease and intestinal lymphomas and other cancers. *Gastroenterology* 128:S79–S86.

Corazza, G.R., Giorgio, Z., Sabatino, A., Ciccocioppo, R. & Gasbarrini, G. (1999) A reassessment of splenic hypofunction in coeliac disease. *The American Journal of Gastroenterology* 94(2):391–397.

Corrao, G., Corazza, G.R., Bagnardi, V., Brusco, G., Ciacci, C., Cottone, M., Satengna Guidetti, C., Usai, P., Cesari, P., Pelli, M., Loperfido, S., Volta, U., Calabrio, A., Certo, M., for the Club del Tenue Study Group (2001) Mortality in patients with coeliac disease and the relatives: A cohort study. *The Lancet* 358:356–361.

Department of Health (1999) *Saving Lives: Our Healthier Nation.* HMSO, London.

Department of Health (2001) *The Expert Patient: A New Approach to Chronic Disease Management for the 21st Century.* HMSO, London.

Department of Health (2004) *Choosing Health. Making Healthy Choices Easier.* HMSO, London.

Goddard, C.J.R. & Gillett, H.R. (2006) Complications of coeliac disease: Are all patients at risk? *Postgraduate Medical Journal* 82:705–712.

Gough, K., Read, A. & Naish, J. (1962) Intestinal reticulosis as a complication of idiopathic steatorrhoea. *Gut* 3:232–239.

Her Majesty's Stationery Office (1996) *Immunisation Against Infectious Diseases.* HMSO, London, pp. 301, 25.1.

Holmes, G.K.T., Prior, P., Lane, M.R., Pope, D. & Allan, R.N. (1989) Malignancy in coeliac disease. Effect of a gluten free diet. *Gut* 30:333–338.

Johnston, S.D. & Robinson, J. (1998) Fatal pneumococcal septicaemia in a coeliac patient. *European Journal of Gastroenterology and Hepatology* 10(4):253–254.

McKay, P.J., Kennedy, D.H. & Lucie, N.P. (1993) Should hyposplenic patients receive prophylaxis against bacterial infection? *Scottish Medical Journal* 38:51–52.

Mckinley, M., Leibowitz, S., Bronzo, R., Zani, I., Weissman, G. & Schiffman, G. (1995) Appropriate response to pneumococcal vaccine in coeliac sprue. *Journal of Clinical Gastroenterology* 20(2):113–116.

Muller, A.F. & Toghill, P.J. (1995) Hyposplenism in gastrointestinal disease. *Gut* 36:165–167.

O'Grady, J.G., Stevens, F.M., Harding, B., Gorman, T., McNicholl, B. & McCarthy, C.F. (1984) Hyposplenism and gluten sensitive enteropathy. Natural history, incidence and relationship to diet and small bowel morphology. *Gastroenterology* 87:1326–1331.

Parnell, N. (1998) Fatal pneumococcal septicaemia in a coeliac patient (Correspondence). *European Journal of Gastroenterology and Hepatology* 10(10):899.

Pietzak, M.M. (2005) Follow up of patients with coeliac disease: Achieving compliance with treatment. *Gastroenterology* 128:S135–S141.

Royal College of Nursing (2006) *Telephone Advice Lines for People Living with Long Term Conditions: Guidance for Nurse Practitioners*. RCN, London.

Shack, L.G., Wood, H.E., Kang, J.Y., Brewster, D.H., Quinn, M.J., Maxwell, J.D. & Majeeds, A. (2006) Small intestinal cancer in England, Wales and Scotland: Time trends in incidence, mortality and survival. *Alimentary Pharmacology and Therapeutics* 23:1297–1306.

Sverker, A., Hensing, G. & Hallert, C. (2005) 'Controlled by food' – lived experiences of coeliac disease. *Journal of Human Nutrition and Dietetics* 18(3):171–180.

Sverker, A., Ostlund, G., Hallert, C. & Hensing, G. (2007) Sharing life with a gluten-intolerant person- the perspective of close relatives. *Journal of Human Nutrition and Dietetics* 20:412–422.

Toofany, S. (2007) Learning the language of health. *Nursing Management* 14(6):10–14.

Walters, J.R.F. (2007) Analysis of the absolute risk in coeliac disease indicates the importance of the prevention of osteoporosis. *Gut* 56(2):310.

West, J., Logan, R.F.A., Smith, C.J., Hubbard, R.B. & Card, T.R. (2004) Malignancy and mortality in people with coeliac disease: Population based cohort study. *British Medical Journal* 329:716–719.

Wright, D.H. (1995) The major complications of coeliac disease. *Bailliere's Clinical Gastroenterology* 9(2):351–369.

Chapter 7
The Impact of Coeliac Disease
and Vulnerable Groups

LEARNING OUTCOMES

At the end of this chapter you should be able to:

- Discuss the emotional impact of coeliac disease at key life stages, namely adolescence, pregnancy and old age.
- Describe how each of these phases is managed.
- Discuss how nurses can help to support the impact during each of these phases.
- Discuss other key phases that might lead to significant challenges in the management of coeliac disease.

Research has found (Ciacci *et al.*, 2002) that patients are often relieved when they receive a diagnosis of coeliac disease, especially after prolonged periods with unexplained symptoms and general ill health. However, patients who have not previously experienced what they would term as ill health describe confusion, distress and anger when diagnosed.

The impact of diagnosis depends not only on their symptoms but also on other factors such as age at diagnosis, family support, their role in society, relationships and even concomitant illness. As these factors change over time so unsurprisingly are there changes in the coping mechanisms that may affect dietary compliance. It is important to be aware of the impact of diagnosis on all groups and in particular vulnerable groups at key stages.

This chapter with the help of case studies looks at some of the challenges faced by patients at and in the years following diagnosis, from adolescence to old age. The aim is to underline the need for continued support and follow-up and give practical advice as to how nurses can help support people during these stages.

EMOTIONAL IMPACT

It is important to take the psychological and social aspects of coeliac disease into account when a diagnosis is made. Studies (Sverker *et al.*, 2005) have shown that the lived experiences of coeliac disease are varied and profound. They describe specific emotions of:

- Isolation
- Shame
- Fear of being contaminated by gluten
- Concerns about being a 'bother'

Most of these issues relate to food as a social priority and, if we think about it, how often do we go out socialising with friends and family without food forming some part of that social life? These emotions often lead to people shunning invitations and becoming virtual recluses, or avoiding disclosing that they have the disease and eating what is offered despite an awareness of the risks. Even within the family environment it is often a battleground when trying to feed an entire family only one of whom has coeliac disease. It is not unknown for partners to withhold housekeeping money on the premise that coeliac foods are too expensive and yet expect to be fed a 'decent' meal themselves.

If we look at our general use and abuse of junk food and the links to obesity, these issues are often not taken seriously despite the obvious risks highlighted by constant media reporting. Why then should we expect a non-coeliac population to understand the risks of gluten ingestion on a sub-clinical disease? Perhaps, a more apt question is 'how do we ensure that a non-coeliac population understands'? Here the role of the nurse can at least indirectly help to reduce the negative social consequences by offering ongoing support, education and information.

ADOLESCENCE

Adolescence is a cultural and social phenomenon as well as a phase of development. It is conventionally seen as that period somewhere between childhood and adulthood from 11 to 18 years, a period where parents of teenage children are often heard either shouting or sighing heavily. For the adolescent it is no picnic either. According to the psychologist Erikson (1950), physical changes lead the young person to become more concerned with their appearance as they strive to develop an identity, often feeling uncomfortable in their new bodies. Socially, they are still dependent on their parents but are expected to behave like adults. Psychologically, they experience the conflicts of adolescence, fluctuating constantly between co-operation and rebellion. Erikson (1950) describes this as a psychosocial crisis of identity versus role confusion. Who am I and what is my goal in life?

On top of this the individual with coeliac disease then starts to explore their underlying chronic disease as a part of their identity – a disease that as a sub-clinical condition is often misunderstood by their peers because it is 'unseen' and therefore does not share the obvious impact of other chronic diseases, like the diabetic forgetting to take their insulin or the asthmatic forgetting to bring their inhalers. Sverker *et al.* (2005) found that when adult individuals who were diagnosed with coeliac disease as children were asked to recount their most recent dilemmas associated with living with the disease they recounted incidents related to their adolescent years as opposed to either childhood or adult years.

When adolescents focus on the condition of coeliac disease to the detriment of their other qualities, there is a risk that they will develop a negative identity. The difficulties experienced in the social arena appear to become more acute when adolescents start socialising with their peer groups more than their families and are faced with the decision of disclosing their 'condition' or pretending it does not exist and going with the flow. Factors that contribute to dietary non-compliance in adolescence include peer pressure, experimentation with alcohol, new partnerships and fear of social exclusion. Tremendous amounts of reassurance along with constant reinforcement of messages around dietary compliance are needed to avoid the consequences of this transitional period.

If adolescents manage to rise above the question of 'who am I' successfully, they still have issues surrounding their goal in life. Here many problems are encountered due to ignorance of employers of the condition. Currently in the United Kingdom, individuals with coeliac disease are excluded from joining the armed forces. If someone with special dietary requirements on religious grounds can join then it does beg the question, why cannot people with coeliac disease? Does it really make them medically unfit to serve? Or is the risk actually greater with those individuals who enter the forces undiagnosed? The police force also appeared to be imposing similar restrictions, but the Home Office Police Recruitment Centre has stated that applications for the police would not be rejected on the grounds of having coeliac disease but taken on individual merit.

There are probably many other areas of employment where similar restrictions are applied but more covertly than the armed forces.

Activity

Look at the key employers in your area. What restrictions do they apply with regard to coeliac disease? If they do, what is their rationale?

For an adolescent with coeliac disease trying to carve out a career, these rejections can have a devastating long-term effect. Legislation that may prove helpful includes the *Single Equality Scheme 2007–2010* (Department of Health, 2007). This is a public commitment from the Department of Health as to how it intends to meet the responsibilities placed on it by equality legislation. As a public document it is answerable to the public for the commitments it sets out. The scheme is based around six equality strands (race, gender, disability, age, sexual orientation, religion and belief) and is also part of the human rights programme. Long-standing illness has previously been categorised as a disability (Department of Health, 2006) and therefore the blanket exclusion of coeliac patients on these grounds may well be challenged before long on the grounds of discrimination.

As the document continues to be updated it will be interesting to follow the long-term commitment to 'equality' for those with long-term illness.

Activity

Familiarise yourself with the single equity scheme. What do you think are its possible applications for those with long-standing illness and in particular coeliac disease?

In addition to the private battles of adolescence, from a medical perspective this is the stage at which their care should transfer from paediatricians to gastroenterologists. Transitional care arrangements vary, but are often quite poor and the biggest risk is of this group falling through the gaps and being lost to follow-up entirely at a time when they are probably at their most vulnerable. Specialist nurses should look at these arrangements and do what they can to ensure a seamless transfer of care. These arrangements will include the challenges of building supportive relationships within a new healthcare environment and team and dealing with the challenges inevitably made to the diagnosis. Although family involvement remains important this is also a time when these youngsters need the space to explore the issues surrounding their identity and role as coeliac patients, independently and in confidence. This can inevitably lead to conflict between parents and the healthcare profession. Not an easy time, but if done sensitively the long-term health effects of good dietary compliance will be seen. Case study 7.1 highlights one such example where despite good transitional care arrangements the challenges to both identity and role led to difficulties in providing adequate follow-up and support. By ensuring that good-quality services supporting the long-term care and follow-up of patients with coeliac disease are universal and not dependent on post-code, then we can at least ensure that adolescents falling by the wayside have a good chance of being picked up again whether as part of a routine medical checkup or as the result of an episode of ill health requiring medical intervention.

Case study 7.1

A 15-year-old boy under the care of the paediatricians since his diagnosis of coeliac disease as a baby had for some years been interested in becoming a pilot in the RAF. With no ill health, a good dietary compliance and a keen rugby player he was devastated to discover that he could not join the RAF because of his coeliac disease. As his diagnosis was made when he was a baby and therefore not within his recollection he challenged the diagnosis. The paediatrician sought advice from the gastroenterologists; it was decided to undertake a further gastroscopy with duodenal biopsies following a gluten challenge and the issue of transferring his care over to the gastroenterology team was discussed and agreed. A further gastroscopy with duodenal biopsies was undertaken following a 2-week gluten challenge, with a minimum daily gluten intake of 10 g (equivalent to four slices of bread). The histology concurred with the original diagnosis of coeliac disease. The nurse endoscopist undertaking the procedure also ran the coeliac follow-up clinic and so was able to see both mum and patient with the news. Obviously, he was very disappointed but there was a promise made to support him if he wanted to challenge the RAF on their decision on an individual basis. The discussion of transferring his care to adult services was concluded and as the assessment showed good dietary compliance, annual telephone follow-up was agreed. Over the course of the next 18 months, there was evidence to suggest that there was an increasing non-compliance with his diet. He was even caught on one occasion by the nurse specialist drinking beer on a night out! Follow-up became more difficult, with each telephone appointment cancelled. It became difficult to pin him down, although he did attend the surgery for the blood tests when sent the forms. Eventually, the ball was put back into his court regarding ongoing follow-up. Although this approach risked him being lost to follow-up, it was necessary that having been transferred to adult care he should be allowed to make a decision regarding his personal health. This was, however, done with the confidence that he had the knowledge about the disease needed to reach that decision.

FERTILITY AND PREGNANCY

Infertility, as discussed in Chapter 3, has been one of the least reported non-gastrointestinal manifestations of coeliac disease and may itself be one of the first clinical symptoms of sub-clinical disease (Eliakim & Sherer, 2001). It has been shown (Collins *et al.*, 1996) that the frequency of positive serology to coeliac disease amongst infertile women is more than ten times that of the general population, indicating that coeliac disease should be considered as a cause in all women with unexplained infertility. Martinellia *et al.* (2000) found a 1:80 prevalence rate of coeliac disease in women screened during pregnancy and also suggested an unfavourable outcome in individuals not following a gluten free diet, including abortion, premature delivery, small birth rate and intrauterine growth retardation. However, a short report submitted by the same group on a larger population sample in 2004 (Greco *et al.*, 2004), whilst showing the same prevalence rate, showed no unfavourable outcome of pregnancy.

It would appear that adhering to a gluten free diet reduces the chances of an adverse pregnancy-related outcome. This highlights the need for early diagnosis to enhance fertility and a favourable pregnancy to term.

Pregnancy, in addition to uncovering previously undiagnosed disease, can at times cause the reactivation of previously quiescent disease, or deterioration of known disease and additional support during pregnancy is important in this group.

Evidence (Greco *et al.*, 2004) suggests that after 12 months on a gluten free diet most women diagnosed with coeliac disease will enjoy a successful pregnancy, nutritional status being better able to support fertility. Therefore, women trying to conceive inside of that 12-month period need to be aware of the increased risks and followed up more closely during the period up to conception.

Another issue to consider is folate intake. Folate is a water-soluble vitamin needed as a daily dietary intake as it cannot be stored in the body. Adults need 0.2 mg a day. The most usual cause of folate deficiency in the Western Hemisphere is inadequate dietary intake. The most common factor precipitating folate deficiency throughout the world is pregnancy, but another major cause of deficiency is coeliac disease (Haslem & Probert, 1998; Hoffbrand, 1971). Therefore, it is reasonable to assume that a coeliac patient poorly compliant with their gluten free diet and trying to conceive has a high risk of failing to conceive or if successful of complications associated with low folate levels, the main one being neural tube defects such as spina bifida. A good dietary intake of folate should be encouraged and this includes green vegetables such as brussel sprouts, broccoli, asparagus and peas. It also includes chickpeas and brown rice and some fruit especially oranges and bananas. Cereals and bread are another good source, but are of course limited foodstuffs to coeliac sufferers. Limited alcohol consumption is also recommended during conception as well as pregnancy as it too adversely affects the absorption and utilisation of folate.

The synthetic pharmaceutical form of folate used for food fortification and in supplements is folic acid, which is more stable in comparison to other forms of the vitamin. In 2000, the Committee on the Medical Aspects of Food Policy (COMA) advised that universal fortification of flour with folic acid would have a significant effect in preventing neural tube defect affected conceptions and births (Department of Health, 2000). The health departments and the Food Standards Agency undertook a public consultation which raised concerns that mandatory fortification of flour with folic acid may mask vitamin B12 deficiency which if untreated could lead to neurological damage, a particular concern in the elderly. This view was upheld by health ministers (Department of Health, 2004a) who agreed that the mandatory fortification of flour was not the way forward. However, they did release a publication information leaflet later in 2004 (Department of Health, 2004b) advising a supplementary dose of folic acid, 0.4 mg daily through conception until the twelfth week of pregnancy. Higher doses of folic acid 5 mg a day may well be needed for those at higher risk (Hoffbrand, 1971), i.e. individuals with coeliac disease. It is important therefore that in addition to a thorough assessment, reassessment of nutrient levels, and importantly B12, and folate levels is made.

Although uncommon in women conceiving under the age of 30 years; as peak bone density is not reached until that age where individuals with coeliac disease and osteoporosis are being treated with bisphosphonates, these have a tetrogenic effect lasting for up to 2 years after stopping the drug. Women of childbearing age should have been warned of this risk prior to commencing these drugs but once taking need to be fully aware of the time lag between stopping the drug and attempting conception.

Routine follow-up is part and parcel of pregnancy and adding the burden of additional follow-up for coeliac disease may not be appropriate. There are as yet no specific guidelines for pregnant women with coeliac disease but continued adherence to a gluten free diet is obviously imperative. An in-depth assessment of dietary compliance, needs and particular stressors early on in the pregnancy will help to identify the level of support needed. There are as we have seen additional concerns surrounding nutrition during pregnancy. It is after all not just the woman's health but potentially the health of her baby that is at stake. Pregnant women regardless of whether or not they have coeliac disease will need and want additional information on what they should and should not eat and drink, whether they should take dietary supplements, safe levels of weight gain etc.

Activity

What are the dietary 'dos and don'ts' during pregnancy (i.e. cheese, pate). Look at the restrictions and recommendations; what are the implications for the coeliac patient trying to balance good nutritional intake with dietary restrictions?

Additional follow-up of the coeliac disease during pregnancy should be based on an initial thorough assessment and then the ongoing needs of the individual. It may simply mean that obstetric follow-up needs to include continued assessment of calcium, iron and vitamin B12 levels with supplementation where necessary. It may be that more intensive dietetic support is required at intervals throughout the duration of the pregnancy. The availability of helpline advice services and telephone follow-up clinics in coeliac disease greatly reduces the burden of additional hospital visits during pregnancy whilst still providing ongoing support to ensure a successful pregnancy. Close follow-up should continue following the birth of the child as balancing a new baby with other family commitments can all lead to additional stress and lapses in dietary compliance.

THE OLDER COELIAC PATIENT

As has already been highlighted the diagnosis of coeliac disease now often occurs much later in life, reportedly comprising up to 25% of the total numbers of patients diagnosed in some centres (Freeman *et al.*, 2002), and patients in their seventies, eighties and even nineties suddenly find themselves having to radically change their lifestyle. Although not insurmountable it does bring its own unique set of issues. The clinical presentations in this age group are influenced to some extent by the long-standing course of the sub-clinical disease before diagnosis. Weight loss and diarrhoea are still commonly reported presentations in the older age group but equally notable is iron deficiency anaemia. In either case this normally results in elderly patients being investigated for colonic malignancy initially, without excluding the possibility of coeliac disease until much later.

Older patients, as with adolescents, may be more likely to challenge the diagnosis. If they have lived this long without any problems, why should they worry about it now at their age? This is especially so if they are asymptomatic at diagnosis. Long-term side effects, even malignancy, are often not as important to an older patient, 'I've had a good innings', so current health gains and the management of immediate risks need to be the initial focus of education with this patient group. However, the number of potentially serious disorders that may complicate the clinical course of the disease in older patients is significant. The delay in diagnosis into older life increases the risk of established associated autoimmune diseases, of small bowel lymphomas (Al-toma *et al.*, 2007) and of metabolic bone disease in particular reduction in bone density (osteopenia/osteoporosis) (Freeman *et al.*, 2002).

Older patients need much closer assessment at diagnosis. Measurement of serum thyroid-stimulating hormone, small bowel follow through, and DEXA scan are imperatives and pneumococcal vaccine should be considered in all older coeliac patients (Freeman *et al.*, 2002).

Concentrating on correcting any nutritional imbalance is vital and here dietetic review is particularly important in addition to measuring serum levels of iron, folate, B12 and fat-soluble vitamins. Unlike younger age groups, they may require some initial supplementation/replacement therapies but these should not be necessary in the long term. Older people normally eat much healthier and more balanced diets having not been bought up on a diet of junk food. This makes it easier in terms of staple dietary foods such as meat and vegetables, but may be more difficult when having to source alternatives to gluten-containing products that mean some experimentation. Age-related deterioration in physical health such as eyesight or manual dexterity can have an impact on everyday taken for granted activities such as reading labels or cooking. Difficulties can be more pronounced when individuals are widowed. Frequently cooking for one has become a chore. Their diet may already be poor or they may have become reliant on ready meals or meals on wheels. Careful assessment is needed without being either patronising or confrontational. A visit by a community dietitian may be useful to assess the home situation; in addition, it is often easier than making frequent pilgrimages into hospital, allowing a more patient-focused assessment. A home visit can answer the questions as to whether there are adequate storage and cooking facilities, what types of foodstuffs are in evidence in the kitchen. Are they connected to utilities such as gas or electricity?

A reduction in bone mineral density is not unusual in this patient group. Treatment should include appropriate lifestyle advice in addition to dietary supplementation of calcium and vitamin D and the more specific therapies. Weight-bearing exercise is still essential, obviously taking into consideration age-related and health restrictions. Walking, gardening and dancing are examples of activities that in addition to improving bone health and making people feel better, rejuvenate muscle tissue and therefore muscle strength, improving coordination and balance.

Follow-up in this age group should be tailored to meet the individual need. Telephone follow-up may be restricted due to poor hearing, although some prefer that method of contact and simply get a family member to sit in with them for the consultation. For some making a visit to the hospital is a way of getting out and having someone to talk to. It may be more suitable for primary care to take over their follow-up, and these services will be discussed in a later chapter. Case study 7.2 outlines one such package of care and underlines the need for careful initial observation and assessment.

Activity

Read Case study 7.2. Map out this gentleman's pathway of care from the case. Can you see any areas where earlier input from different care agencies might have made a difference? What agencies would you have used?

Case study 7.2

A 77-year-old gentleman was referred for investigation of iron deficiency anaemia and found to have coeliac disease. All baseline investigations were normal apart from his DEXA scan showing osteopenia.

At presentation following diagnosis, he was found to be quite frail and unkempt with a variety of safety pins and staples holding the hem up on his trousers. He was a widower living alone but very independent, managing his own cooking and shopping and regularly walking the mile in and out of town. His nearest relatives lived in Yorkshire. A community dietetic review was undertaken to look more closely at his home environment and this appeared satisfactory. He was very keen to get to grips with a gluten free diet and even attended a number of local coeliac group cookery demonstrations, although because of poor hearing he struggled to take in all of the information. Nevertheless, he left the meetings with a carrier bag full of gluten free 'goodies' to try. Despite his apparent frailty his fierce independence meant that he considered free prescriptions of 'food' as charity and insisted on buying his bread, flour etc. at obviously great expense. It took regular persuasion from the hospital and GP before he finally agreed to have his entitlement of gluten free foods on prescription. He loved coming into outpatients for a 'chat', so hospital review was continued initially on a 6 monthly basis because of his frailty and also some ongoing anaemia. Five years after diagnosis he suffered a mild stroke, further exacerbating his frailty. At clinic, he was noted to be losing weight and had become quite tearful. He also reported some altered bowel habit. Bloods showed a worsening anaemia but also abnormal LFTs. He underwent a series of investigations over the next 12 months including barium enema, abdominal ultrasound and CT scan. These investigations punctuated by a stay in hospital after a fall and a spell in a residential care home from where it was decided that he needed more home support and therefore moved to a warden-controlled flat in the city centre. He continued to be reviewed in outpatients at regular intervals and although tearful valued the support of familiar faces. At his last clinic appointment, he had moved into his warden-controlled flat and was getting gluten free meals from the WRVS who also spent a little time with him each day and left him frozen meals for the weekend. He had managed to put on some weight and although still experiencing some diarrhoea this was now very intermittent. His bloods improved although were not back to normal and continue to be monitored, although investigations have excluded any underlying pathology.

This chapter has highlighted just three specific areas where individuals with coeliac disease are possibly more vulnerable in terms of accepting and adhering to a gluten free diet and therefore the risks associated with non-compliance. Obviously, there are many stages between those mentioned at which a coeliac patient may become more vulnerable; setting up home within a new relationship, bereavement, divorce, concomitant diagnosis or serious illness etc.; the list is endless. This reinforces the need for ongoing flexible follow-up.

HINTS AND TIPS

- Discuss with colleagues how transitional care from children's to adult services will be managed. Consider initially sitting in on the consultations with the paediatric teams so that the child becomes familiar with the adult team. Perhaps offer to start to provide telephone support between clinic appointments. Think about the provision of other support networks, local groups, buddies etc.

- Draft a template letter to potential employers to support patients in gaining employment. Remember to offer employers information and education too, as often they are ignorant of the implications of having the disease and imagine instant 'collapse' if employees with coeliac disease as much as eat gluten.
- Think about how you will support women with coeliac disease in both the conception phase and during pregnancy. Look at shared care arrangements, frequency and modality of follow-up.
- Ensure that you include a careful history of the social circumstances when assessing and following up the older patient with coeliac disease. Source the network support that you might need to make referral to, i.e. social services, housing etc.

REFERENCES

Al-toma, A., Verbeek, W.H.M., Hadithi, M., von Blomberg, B.M.E. & Mulder, C.J.J. (2007) Survival in refractory coeliac disease and enteropathy-associated T-cell lymphoma: Retrospective evaluation of single-centre experience. *Gut* 56:1373–1378.

Ciacci, C., Iavarone, A., Siniscalchi, M., Romano, R. & De Rosa, A. (2002) Psychological dimensions of coeliac disease. *Digestive Disease Science* 47:2082–2087.

Collins, P., Vilska, S., Heinoen, P.K., Hallstrom, O. & Pikkarainen, P. (1996) Infertility and coeliac disease. *Gut* 39: 382–384.

Department of Health (2000) *Folic Acid and the Prevention of Disease. Report on Health and Social Subjects 50*. HMSO, London.

Department of Health (2004a) *Health Ministers Decision on the Fortification of Flour with Folic Acid* (Letter). HMSO, London. http://www.dh.gov.uk/en/publicationsandstatistics/letter sandcirculars/dearcolleagueletters/dh_4085302. Accessed 15 August 2007.

Department of Health (2004b) *Thinking of Having a Baby: Folic Acid – an Essential Ingredient in Making Babies.*

HMSO, London. http://www.dh.gov.uk/en/publication/ publicationpolicyandguidance/dh_4081396. Accessed 15 August 2007.

Department of Health (2006) *Creating a Disability Equality Scheme: Guidance for the NHS.* HMSO, London.

Department of Health (2007) *Single Equality Scheme: 2007–2010.* HMSO, London.

Eliakim, R. & Sherer, D.M. (2001) Coeliac disease: Fertility and pregnancy. *Gynecologic and Obstetric Investigation* 51:3–7.

Erikson, E.H. (1950) *Childhood and Society.* Norton, New York.

Freeman, H., Lemoyne, M. & Pare, P. (2002) Coeliac disease. *Best Practice and Research Clinical Gastroenterology* 16(1):37–49.

Greco, L., Veneziano, A., Di Donato, L., Zampella, C., Pecoraro, M., Paladini, D., Paparo, F., Vollaro, A. & Marinelli, P. (2004) Undiagnosed coeliac disease does not appear to be associated with unfavourable outcome of pregnancy. *Gut* 53:149–151.

Haslem, N. & Probert, C. (1998) An audit of the investigation and treatment of folic acid deficiency. *Journal of the Royal Society of Medicine* 91:72–73.

Hoffbrand, A.V. (1971) Folate absorption. *Journal of Clinical Pathology* 24(5):66–76.

Martinellia, P., Troncone, R., Paparo, F., Torre, P., Trapanese, E., Fasano, C., Lamberti, A., Budillon, G., Nardone, G. & Greco, L. (2000) Coeliac disease and unfavourable outcome in pregnancy. *Gut* 46:332–335.

Sverker, A., Hensing, G. & Hallert, C. (2005) 'Controlled by food' – lived experiences of coeliac disease. *Journal of Human Nutrition and Dietetics* 18(3):171–180.

Chapter 8
Managing Poor Response or Relapse

LEARNING OUTCOMES

At the end of this chapter you should be able to:

- Discuss the definition of refractory disease and the associated risks.
- Describe the assessment process of those with poor dietary response or relapse.
- List the concomitant conditions that should be excluded as a cause of poor response or relapse.
- Describe the strategies for managing poor response.

Individuals with coeliac disease can continue to have or redevelop symptoms despite being on a gluten free diet, the most frequent symptom being diarrhoea. The commonest cause is lack of adherence to a gluten free diet, either deliberate or accidental, but there are other reasons and persistent symptoms should be investigated exactly as you would in a patient without coeliac disease.

This chapter builds on the previous chapters and together with its case study highlights the importance of ongoing support and follow-up and is central in underlining the need to exclude concomitant disease or complications and not rely wholly on the assumption that dietary indiscretions are always the cause.

Case study 8.1

A 49-year-old single gentleman referred originally with a 6-month history of diarrhoea, weight loss and abdominal discomfort. He was known to have type 2 diabetes with a degree of peripheral neuropathy; there was a history of previous episodes of diarrhoea thought to be due to irritable bowel syndrome. There was a family history of diabetes but none of coeliac disease. He was a non-smoker, denied any alcohol intake and had recently been made redundant adding to his anxieties. With a positive EMA it was likely that he had coeliac disease; however, he was reluctant to undergo endoscopy and so initially was put on a gluten free diet by his GP and referred to the dietitians. Whilst there was some improvement he continued to suffer with diarrhoea up to nine times a day. He eventually agreed to an endoscopy with sedation, following reintroduction of a gluten-containing diet. This confirmed the diagnosis of coeliac disease with Marsh grade 3b changes. In view of his diabetes and peripheral neuropathy there was also the question of autonomic diarrhoea related to bile salt malabsorption and it was also arranged for him to have a SeCHAT test; this was negative. He was therefore advised to continue with his gluten free diet but in addition a lactose-free diet in case of secondary lactose intolerance. He was followed up closely by the dietitians over the next few months who confirmed, with the help of his food diary, good compliance with his gluten free diet. It was noted that his diabetic control was worsening and he continued to have what he described as 'explosive' diarrhoea and persistent weight loss. He was given loperamide to use as symptomatic relief. Obviously, the severity of his symptoms and resultant lethargy was preventing him from finding another job, adding to the anxiety. Living alone meant that he had no immediate support from family or friends. He went on to have a baseline DEXA scan and small bowel follow-through, both of which were normal.

Seven months following the histological diagnosis of coeliac disease he continued to have diarrhoea up to six times a day and so underwent a further endoscopy and duodenal biopsies, which showed improvement with *regeneration of some of the villi*.

He remained very symptomatic and at review 4 months following his endoscopy reported worsening diarrhoea up to 20 times a day. At this point, his diabetic medication was reviewed as a cause and despite negative SeCHAT a trial of cholestyramine was suggested. These strategies were both unsuccessful making no impact on the diarrhoea. A stool collection for faecal fat was taken, which showed a slight excess of fat in the stool. In the first instance an enteroscopy was arranged and undertaken 8 months after the previous endoscopy. Histology on this occasion showed a vast improvement and was reported as Marsh 1 *consistent with coeliac disease being managed on a gluten free diet.* His symptoms continued and it was noted at follow-up 3 months later that he was compulsively drinking up to 6 L of water a day, which it was felt could be contributing. He underwent a water deprivation test but despite this the diarrhoea continued. In view of the slight excess increase of fat in the stool, a faecal elastane ELISA was arranged and this showed a borderline low reading. Although not clearly diagnostic of exocrine pancreatic insufficiency at the time of writing a trial of Creon, supplements had been suggested.

PERSISTENT DISEASE

A small minority of individuals with coeliac disease will suffer with persistent symptoms that do not improve on a gluten free diet; others will relapse some time after a seemingly good initial dietary response. Some of these will be found to have refractory disease defined as continued or recurrent malabsorption and diarrhoea associated with persisting moderate or severe villous atrophy despite strict adherence to a gluten free diet (AGA, 2006; Daum *et al.*, 2005). Refractory coeliac disease can be controlled with systemic corticosteroids/immunosuppressants leading to a rapid cessation of symptoms. However, there is a noticeable deterioration in health again within days of stopping treatment and because of this they are thought best avoided (BSG, 2002), especially until other causes of poor response have been excluded. There is also cohort of refractory patients who will fail to respond to any treatments, including immunosuppression. Immunologically, there are different types of refractory coeliac disease that will account for this (Al-toma *et al.*, 2007). It is the latter group that are thought to be at highest risk of developing enteropathy T-cell lymphoma.

Individuals with coeliac disease should, however, be reassured that in the majority of cases there is a satisfactory clinical and histological response to a gluten free diet and it is only a small minority 2–8% (Daum *et al.*, 2005; Howdle, 1991) that fail to respond.

According to the British Society of Gastroenterology (2002), the assessment of patients with coeliac disease who fail to respond to a gluten free diet involves three steps:

1. Assessment of dietary compliance
2. Confirmation of the diagnosis
3. Exclusion of concomitant disease

As highlighted in previous chapters, the aims of the initial assessment and continued follow-up are, in principle, to ensure all three steps. In the case of continued poor response this becomes more rigorous to exclude concomitant disease such as microscopic colitis, bacterial overgrowth, giardiasis, lactose intolerance, pancreatic exocrine insufficiency, small bowel strictures, small bowel lymphomas and other gastrointestinal malignancies.

The effect on these patients can of course be devastating. They are interrogated as to their dietary compliance and then they are faced with the possibility of further investigations challenging their diagnosis or looking for other illnesses. In some cases, they remain extremely unwell with chronic fatigue – a key symptom. Sensitivity and clear and honest information is an imperative, ensuring that they remain fully informed of the outcomes of all tests and investigations in a timely manner.

ASSESSMENT OF DIETARY COMPLIANCE

Very often here, dietary lapses are unintentional due to particularly resistant disease or as a result of a large area of affected small intestine. Highly symptomatic patients will recognise immediately when they have ingested gluten and it is then easier to identify the source. Patients who were previously asymptomatic or whose symptoms have never settled on their diet will find it more difficult to pinpoint the source. Assessment needs to look extremely closely at the diet and involve frequent trained dietetic input. In addition to a thorough review of their diet, having a food diary analysed by the dietitians is particularly useful; attention needs to be paid to:

- Are they eating previously 'safe' foods that now due to a change in manufacturing processes have become 'unsafe' Recheck all foods that have been regularly consumed and are not labelled specifically as 'gluten free'.
- Have all medications been checked, in particular medications or supplements bought over the counter. Gluten is used as a filler in pill capsules (Freeman *et al.*, 2002).
- Are they eating oats? Despite the contention regarding their safety, people with resistant disease may be sensitive to even very low levels of contaminant, and these should be excluded from the diet until there is a satisfactory clinical response.
- Is there a risk of cross-contamination? Even with the greatest care there is always the risk of cross-contamination, both in and out of the home (see section 'Exclusion of Concomitant Disease'). Given the different levels of sensitivity, additional advice should be given to avoid the risks where possible (Table 8.1).
- Are they drinking alcohol containing gluten? Alcohol may contain clinically significant quantities of gluten and often patients as well as clinicians forget this (Sussman *et al.*, 2007). Beers, lagers, ales and stouts should be excluded unless specifically gluten free. Wines, ciders, liqueurs and spirits are generally safe to consume but caution should be exercised when mixing drinks or buying drinks 'pre-mixed' that the mixer does not contain gluten. Some wine coolers for example may be malt based. Also, some ciders may add barley for enzymes and flavour.

Activity

List a selection of alcoholic drinks including mixed drinks, i.e. gin and tonic. Which contain gluten? How easy is it to find gluten free beers?

Table 8.1   Additional advice to those with apparent resistant disease

Advice	Rationale
• It may be necessary to have your own area of the kitchen with separate cooking utensils and cupboards to store your food.	• Even dust from gluten free products, i.e. cereal packets, is a potential source of contamination.
• Do not use wooden cooking utensils; use metal or plastic.	• Gluten contaminates wooden utensils, which becomes ingrained and is not easily removed by washing.
• Similarly use glass rather than wooden chopping boards.	• As above.
• Do not eat from any dips etc. where others are also dipping gluten-containing foods, such as crisps or crackers.	• Potential source of contamination.
• Be aware of breadcrumbs on the butter/jam/marmalade.	• As above.
• When using your barbeque, always cook your food first and on a thoroughly cleaned surface.	• Cooking/burning does not destroy gluten, so if food (i.e. beef burger) is cooked before yours, it will be contaminated.
• Do not kiss the children/partner/relative/friend if they have just been eating a wheat-based cereal.	• Potential source of contamination.
• When eating out, seek advice from outlets as to potential sources of contamination and beware of seemingly 'safe' foods.	• Some foods are stored, prepared or even partially cooked alongside gluten-containing foods. Some safe foods such as jacket potato and grated cheese may not be safe if the cheese is bought ready grated as flour is often used to keep the grains separate.

- Is there any untreated nutritional deficiency? – that is, zinc, magnesium, B12, folate. Or have they a lactose intolerance as a result of mucosal atrophy, in which case a trial of low lactose or lactose-free diet with review after 4 weeks may be beneficial (Travis *et al.*, 2005)?

Very often dietary indiscretions are small and totally accidental; however, occasionally closer questioning will reveal deliberate non-compliance. The nursing role in this instance is to elicit the underlying cause and try to provide the appropriate education and support pointing to a strict adherence to a gluten free diet as having a protective effect on the occurrence of malignancy as a long-term risk.

CONFIRMATION OF DIAGNOSIS

Once the gluten free diet has been formally assessed for non-compliance or inadvertent consumption then the next step is in confirming the original diagnosis. The first stage is to review the diagnostic pathway.

- What were the presenting symptoms leading up to the diagnosis?
- Were the investigations undertaken at the time appropriate to the presenting symptoms?
- Was the diagnosis made on the basis of serological markers alone?
- Was the histological finding clear or ambiguous?
- Was there an initial response to the gluten free diet; if yes, at what point following diagnosis did the symptoms deteriorate?

It is worth revisiting the initial history to see what the presenting symptoms were. This should be done in conjunction with a review of the investigations undertaken at the time. For example, if the patient was referred with iron deficiency anaemia, were large bowel investigations carried out to exclude coexistent large bowel pathology or malignancy? We often forget that individuals can have more than one pathology, and this is especially true of coeliac patients where other autoimmune conditions are known to coexist as has been discussed in earlier chapters.

Where patients are reluctant to have an endoscopy to confirm the diagnosis it is possible that sole reliance is placed on the serological test. As has been shown serological markers have different sensitivities and specificities, dependent not only on the commercial test used and its interpretation but also on the geographical and genetic population on which it is used, and therefore should not be used as the sole criterion for making a diagnosis of coeliac disease or indeed in checking for a dietary response in resistant disease. Other investigation modalities such as capsule endoscopy should be considered in apparent resistant disease, if the individual's fears regarding endoscopy cannot be allayed.

Activity

How would you explain to a person unresponsive to their gluten free diet the need for further/repeat investigation? How would you support them through the process both physically and psychologically?

As with the clinical presentation of coeliac disease there is increasing recognition that the pathologic presentation of the disease also varies. Therefore, the original histology should be revisited. If in doubt, a repeat endoscopy and biopsy is recommended following a gluten challenge, provided that the patient is well enough to tolerate this.

EXCLUSION OF CONCOMITANT DISEASE

The third step, once both diagnosis and dietary compliance have been investigated and confirmed, is in excluding other disease. The symptoms should be investigated just as you would in a patient not diagnosed as having coeliac disease. As Case study 8.1 shows despite investigation, a definitive diagnosis or cause for poor response or relapse cannot always be found. There are a number of diseases that can be superimposed on coeliac disease, including:

- Giardiasis
- Bacterial overgrowth
- Ulcerative jejunoileitis
- Microscopic colitis
- Pancreatic exocrine insufficiency
- Enteropathy-related T-cell lymphoma

Note with each of these the similarity between their predominant symptoms and those of coeliac disease.

Giardiasis

Giardiasis is an intestinal infection affecting about 200 million people worldwide (Travis *et al.*, 2005) and is caused by a microscopic parasite called *Giardia lamblia* which lives in faeces. Giardia is not a bacteria but a protozoa and is one of the most common causes of diarrhoea throughout the world. It is also the most common gut parasite in the United Kingdom affecting children more than adults (NHS Direct, 2007). Although infection is associated with travel abroad it can be acquired in the United Kingdom, but history of recent travel abroad should lead to an increased suspicion. In about 15% of cases individuals will carry the parasite but remain asymptomatic; the remainder will suffer from a range of gastrointestinal symptoms including diarrhoea, abdominal pain, anorexia and nausea. Often symptoms of persistent diarrhoea and weight loss occur after an acute attack of gastroenteritis (Travis *et al.*, 2005). Incubation is between 2 and 3 weeks and transmission is through contaminated water or the faecal–oral route.

Investigations to exclude *Giardia lamblia* include obtaining stool samples, stool specimens to detect the cysts will only detect about 60% of cases and stool ELISA is therefore preferred being 92% sensitive and 98% specific (Travis *et al.*, 2005). Jejunal aspiration or biopsy is the most reliable method of detection but obviously entails a further endoscopic procedure. Treatment is with antibiotics, normally metronidazole 750 mg three times a day for 3 days. Very occasionally, Giardiasis will prove resistant to standard antibiotic treatment; however, reinfection or another disease is more common. As it is easily transmitted, in confirmed cases it is sensible to treat the whole family at the same time to prevent reinfection at a later date. Hygiene advice should be given, including washing hands thoroughly after toileting, before food preparation and after changing any animal litters. Because the cysts can live for some time outside the body, clothing, bedding, towels etc. should be washed and all toilets, baths, sinks including taps, handles etc. should be thoroughly cleaned.

Bacterial overgrowth

The entire gastrointestinal tract, including the small intestine, normally contains bacteria. The number of bacteria is greatest in the colon with at least 1 000 000 000 bacteria per millilitre of fluid and much lower in the small intestine less than 10 000 bacteria per millilitre of fluid. The types of bacteria within the small intestine are different than the types of bacteria within the colon. Bacterial overgrowth occurs when the numbers of bacteria within the small intestine increase to almost the same level as those found in the large bowel. Symptoms include diarrhoea, abdominal pain, bloating, fatigue and in severe cases malabsorption resulting from the bacteria either metabolising nutrients or causing inflammation, hindering their absorption. Causes of bacterial overgrowth include disorders of motility that slow down transit through the gut increasing bacterial concentrations such as diverticula, disorders of the immune system such as the use of immunosuppressants or IgA deficiency and disorders allowing movement of bacteria from the colon into the small bowel. Some medications also have the potential to cause bacterial overgrowth including proton pump inhibitors, as in suppressing stomach acid they affect the antibacterial properties of stomach acid. Diagnosis is similar to that for giardiasis in that jejunal aspiration is the gold standard. Biopsies, however, can histologically mimic coeliac disease, making diagnosis challenging. Hydrogen breath test after lactulose is a non-invasive alternative but has a poor sensitivity and specificity (Travis *et al.*, 2005). Where bacterial overgrowth is suspected small bowel radiology should be undertaken to exclude diverticulosis or strictures. However, if done at baseline on diagnosis of coeliac disease the original investigation will provide the necessary evidence, depending on the time lag between the investigations and the relapse.

Treatment is again by antibiotics, often cyclical for the first week of every month to prevent tolerance, rotating between the key antibiotics, metronidazole, tetracycline and amoxicillin. Probiotics are dietary supplements containing potentially beneficial bacteria or yeasts that are widely available and may alter the bacterial flora of the gut to good effect; however, their role remains uncertain. If an anatomical problem is suggested as a cause then surgical correction might be indicated.

Activity

Look up the evidence for both pro- and prebiotics. What are the differences between the two? What are the sources of each and the benefits and disadvantages of the various products?

Ulcerative jejunoileitis

The BSG (2002) describe this as:

> an unusual complication in which unresponsive coeliac disease is associated with ulceration and stricturing (p. 7).

Many terms are found in the literature to describe this same condition, including ulcerative jejunitis, refractory coeliac disease and refractory sprue. If untreated, the initial mucosal inflammation progresses to produce ulceration and stricturing resulting in irreversible damage and a 'point of no return', after which, response to a gluten free diet is poor or non-existent and patients become increasingly resistant to any form of medical treatment. As a result these patients are often severely ill with ulcerations in the jejunum and ileum – and albeit rarely, in the duodenum – and malignant transformation into a T-cell lymphoma is not uncommon. The difference between ulcerative jejunoileitis and lymphoma can often only be made at surgery (BSG, 2002), making careful investigation imperative. Chronic ulceration and scarring can lead to stricture formation which can mimic the clinical manifestations and endoscopic appearances of Crohn's disease. Investigation is by small bowel radiology or enteroscopy. More recently, wireless capsule endoscopy has successfully been used to diagnose the disease (LePane et al., 2007). With the risk of stricture formation there is also obviously the associated risk of non-passage of the capsule. Although a complication, it is obviously also diagnostic and of those cases reported (LePane et al., 2007) the symptoms have resolved and the capsule passed following treatment with prednisolone. However, the long-term survival for patients with ulcerative jejunoileitis beyond 5 years has been reported (Medicine Net, 2007) as being less than 50%.

Microscopic colitis

Microscopic colitis is an inflammatory disease of the colon that causes chronic diarrhoea as its primary symptom and sometimes abdominal pain experienced by a small minority of coeliac patients. Unlike ulcerative colitis rectal blood loss is unusual. It is termed microscopic because at endoscopy the bowel appears normal to the naked eye (macroscopically), with inflammation visible only when biopsies are viewed microscopically. There are two types of microscopic colitis, lymphocytic and collagenous. In lymphocytic colitis there is, as it sounds, an accumulation of lymphocytes within the lining of the colon seen microscopically. In collagenous colitis, there is an additional layer of collagen giving the appearance of scar tissue. There is some question as to whether the two describe different stages of the same disease process. Certainly in microscopic colitis the otherwise chronic inflammation microscopically shows no evidence of either collagen or intraepithelial lymphocytes (Travis et al., 2005).

Drugs can be the cause in up to half of all reported cases (Travis et al., 2005), so it is important to exclude a drug history when investigating poor response or relapse, especially

non-steroidal anti-inflammatory drugs (NSAIDs) and proton
pump inhibitors (PPIs) used to treat dyspeptic symptoms.
Treatment very much depends on the cause and response. Importantly, NSAIDs and PPIs should be stopped. However, careful consideration should be given to alternative treatments.
Standard 5-amino-saciliyate (5ASA) treatment as used in inflammatory bowel disease will be effective in about half of
all cases as will cholestyramine (Travis *et al.*, 2005). If these
treatment modalities fail or a prompt response is needed then
budesonide is effective in over 75% of cases, although symptoms may relapse on stopping (Medicine Net, 2007). In these
cases despite the paucity of supporting evidence, immunosuppressants such as azathioprine may be considered to control
symptoms unresponsive to other treatments.

Activity

Look up the indications and contraindications for both 5ASAs and
azathioprine.

Pancreatic exocrine insufficiency

Pancreatic exocrine insufficiency is commonly associated with
diseases such as pancreatitis or cystic fibrosis but the association with cocliac disease was first reported as far back as
1957 (Dreiling, 1957). This is a condition in which patients
have a shortage of the digestive enzymes necessary to break
down food and digest the fats, proteins and carbohydrates
contained in food. This leads to the malabsorption of nutrients and associated anorexia, weight loss, abdominal pain and
diarrhoea/steatorrhoea. Steatorrhoea occurs when pancreatic
enzyme secretion is <10% normal (Travis *et al.*, 2005).

Confirming the diagnosis of pancreatic exocrine insufficiency can be clinically difficult. Certainly in the early stages
some of the more indirect tests such as the pancreolauryl
test, although specific, are not sensitive enough (Murray *et al.*,
2003) and direct tests such as endoscopic retrograde cholangiopancreatography (ERCP) are invasive and costly for routine
use. Measurement of faecal pancreatic elastase is convenient

and non-invasive and correlates well with the pancreatic output of elastase-1, a proteolytic enzyme produced specifically by the pancreas and unlike other pancreatic enzymes not degraded in its passage through the gut (Stein *et al.*, 1996). Treatment is with pancreatic enzyme supplements such as Creon® and is normally highly effective. It is important that the capsules are taken at the right time, which is during meals and with plenty of fluids, as a rare side effect is the build-up of uric acid in the blood and urine. A low-fat diet is also important in addition to pancreatic supplements; again dietetic input is vital (Travis *et al.*, 2005). Creon® enzymes are taken from pig pancreas glands and so may not be suitable for those with allergies to pork, vegans or those avoiding pork on religious grounds, i.e. Jews.

Enteropathy-related T-cell lymphoma

There are two types of lymphoma: Hodgkin's and non-Hodgkin's lymphoma. These are further divided into T cell and B cell, depending on whether T lymphocytes or B lymphocytes are involved. Normal T cells co-operate with B cells in a complex manner to provide us with our 'immune system' which is capable of recognising foreign invaders such as bacteria and viruses (Hatton, 2005).

Lymphomas appear to be derived from these normal lymphatic immune cells, cells that have undergone a genetic alteration allowing cancer cells to develop. In addition to the division of lymphomas into T-cell and B-cell types, there is then a further division into subtypes. The categories depend on how the cell types are affected. In the case of coeliac patients the risk is from the subgroup of enteropathy-associated T-cell lymphomas as a result of a proliferation of abnormal intraepithelial T lymphocytes.

The mechanism by which coeliac disease predisposes to lymphoma is unclear. Using flow cytometric immunophenotyping, refractory coeliac disease (RCD) has recently been categorised into two types RCDI and RCDII. RCDI has a normal expression of T-cell surface markers, running a benign course, and RCDII shows an atypical population which has a definite pre-lymphoma potential (Al-toma *et al.*, 2007). It is in the latter group that the risk of developing an enteropathy-associated T-cell lymphoma is greatest, and this group appears to be resistant to known therapies. A recent study (Al-toma *et al.*, 2007) found no coeliac-disease-related mortality in the RCDI group with an overall 5 years' survival of 96% compared with the RCDII group where there was an overall survival of only 58%, 56% dying from coeliac-related diseases, 46% of those enteropathy-related T-cell lymphomas.

It would seem that individuals with enteropathy-related T-cell lymphomas (EATL) (Al-toma *et al.*, 2007) present in two different clinical patterns, those with well-established coeliac disease who deteriorate because of the development of RCDII, presenting with the return of symptoms such as diarrhoea, weight loss and fatigue, or those who develop EATL without a history of complicated coeliac disease, presenting often with perforation or obstruction.

Standard investigations such as small bowel radiology and jejunal biopsy will normally give a low yield, even when the presence of EATL is suspected, probably because of the coexistent villous atrophy (BSG, 2002). Small bowel enteroscopy, wireless video capsule endoscopy and computed tomography scan will give a greater yield, with the final diagnosis coming from either good endoscopic biopsies or full-thickness laparoscopic biopsies (Catassi *et al.*, 2005). Treatment is difficult, involving surgery (certainly when presenting with perforation or obstruction), radiotherapy and chemotherapy. Survival is low, with a 2-year survival reported between 15 and 20% (Al-toma *et al.*, 2007) and a 30-month survival at 12% (Howdle *et al.*, 2003). Further studies are obviously required to define more accurately the cut-off point between acceptably normal and pathologically increased percentages of atypical T cells (Al-toma, 2007) to ensure that those with at the highest risk from refractory coeliac disease can be identified.

What is clear from this chapter is that there are numerous causes for poor disease response or relapse, not all caused by the lack of adherence to a gluten free diet. This underlines once again the need for regular follow-up. However, the criteria for follow-up of patients with coeliac disease is not as well defined or standardised as it is when diagnosing the disease

(Bardella *et al.*, 2007). Is 'response' based on clinical or histological criteria or both? Why it is necessary to bear this in mind is that whilst the symptoms of coeliac disease will disappear quite quickly for most on a gluten free diet, with repeat autoantibodies becoming negative, serological markers have a poor negative predictive value and there are individuals in whom symptoms are absent but in whom histology will show severely damaged intestinal mucosa (Bardella *et al.*, 2007). The risk of these patients going on to develop relapse in the future cannot be ignored and bearing in mind the discussion on the risks of those with RCDII and the identification of pathologically increased percentages of atypical T cells, further work needs to be done to look at how we can improve the early identification and hopefully therefore intervention in this group of coeliac patients. In the interim, we need to be aware of the factors associated with a high risk for the development of EATLs and ensure that patients are supported during any ongoing investigation and treatment.

HINTS AND TIPS

- It is important that a division between nursing and medical roles is agreed, as there will be an inevitable blurring of boundaries. Using the suggested algorithm (Figure 6.1) think about how you will manage those with refractory disease? At what point will you refer back to medical colleagues, if not to take over their care at least for discussion?
- Would the 'boundaries' benefit from the development of a specific pathway of assessment and investigation where there is indication of poor response or relapse?
- Be aware of referral pathways to other specialties to enable prompt referral where concomitant conditions are identified.

REFERENCES

Al-toma, A., Verbeek, W., Hadithi, M., Von Blomberg, B. & Mulder, C. (2007) Survival in refractory coeliac disease and enteropathy-associated T-cell lymphoma: Retrospective evaluation of a single-centre experience. *Gut* 56:1373–1378.

American Gastroenterology Association (2006) Coeliac disease. *Gastroenterology* 131(6):1977–1980.

Bardella, M.T., Velio, P., Cesana, B.M., Prampolini, L., Casella, G., Di Bella, C., Lanzini, A., Gambarotti, M., Bassotti, G. & Villanacci, V. (2007). Coeliac disease: A histological follow-up study. *Histopathology* 50:465–471.

British Society of Gastroenterology (2002) *Guidelines for the Management of Patients with Coeliac Disease.* BSG, London.

Catassi, C., Bearzi, I. & Holmes, G. (2005) Association of celiac disease and intestinal lymphomas and other cancers. *Gastroenterology* 128(4):S79–S86.

Daum, S., Cellier, C. & Mulder, C.J. (2005) Refractory coeliac disease. *Best Practice Research Clinical Gastroenterology* 19:413–424.

Dreiling, D.A. (1957) The pancreatic secretion in the malabsorption syndrome and related malnutrition states. *Journal Mount Sinai Hospital New York* 24:243–250.

Freeman, H., Lemoyne, M. & Pare, P. (2002) Coeliac disease. *Best Practice and Research Clinical Gastroenterology* 16(1):37–49.

Hatton, C. (2005) What are T-cell lymphomas? *Lymphoma Support Group News Letter.* http://www.lymphoma.org.uk/support/newsletter/Autumn%202005/whatareTcelllymphomas.htm. Accessed 23 September 2007.

Howdle, P.D. (1991) Coeliac disease: Therapeutic choices in non-responders to conventional therapy. In G. Dobrillo, K.D. Badhan & A. Stiel (eds), *Non-Responders in Gastroenterology.* Cortina International, Verona, pp. 129–139.

Howdle, P.D., Jalal, P.K., Holmes, G. & Houlston, R. (2003) Primary small bowel malignancy in the U.K. and its association with coeliac disease. *QJM: An International Journal of Medicine* 96:345–353.

LePane, C.A., Barkin, J.S., Parra, J. & Simon, T. (2007) Ulcerative Jejunoileitis: A complication of celiac sprue simulating Crohn's disease diagnosed with capsule endoscopy (pillcam). *Digestive Disease Science* 52:698–701.

Medicine Net (2007) *Celiac Disease.* http://www.medicinenet.com/celiac_disease/page11.htm. Accessed 19 September 2007.

Murray, I.A., Clenton, S., McGeorge, B.A. & Safe, A.F. (2003) Retrospective audit of the value of the pancreolauryl test in a district general hospital. *Postgraduate Medical Journal* 79:471–473.

NHS Direct (2007) *Health Encyclopaedia: Giardiasis.* http://www.nhsdirect.nhs.uk/articles/article.aspx?articleId=174&sectionId=1. Accessed 15 September 2007.

Stein, J., Jung, M., Sziegoleit, A., Zeuzem, S., Caspary, W.F. & Lembcke, B. (1996) Immunoreactive elastase 1: Clinical evaluation of a new non-invasive test of pancreatic function. *Clinical Chemistry* 42:222–226.

Sussman, D.A., Barkin, J. & Barkin, J.S. (2007) Letters to the editor: Diet resistant celiac disease. *American Journal of Gastroenterology* 102(8):1833–1834.

Travis, S.P., Ahmad, T., Collier, J. & Hillary, S. (2005) Small intestine, malabsorption. In *Gastroenterology*. Blackwell publishing, Oxford, pp. 214–235.

Chapter 9
Future Developments

LEARNING OUTCOMES

At the end of this chapter you should be able to:

- Discuss chronic disease management and how it sits within the social and political context of today's healthcare priorities.
- Discuss the importance of a continued awareness into our changing knowledge of coeliac disease.
- Discuss the key current developments into the treatment of coeliac disease.

As coeliac disease is a permanent state of intolerance to gluten, requiring life-long adherence to a gluten free diet, it is classed as a chronic disease, one that can be controlled but not cured. Chronic disease can be a drain on healthcare resources and a social challenge and its impact on the quality of life of the individual enormous. For those with coeliac disease, it is the impact on families and the overall quality of life for the affected individual that can lead to non-adherence to treatment and challenges to the diagnosis, especially when those individuals are symptom free. However, we know the risks of continued exposure to gluten and therefore research has focused on early detection, accurate diagnosis, successful treatment and defining its relationship with other diseases. However in the future, we will see more research centred on topics such as alternatives to the gluten free diet and even potential 'cures'.

At some point following diagnosis the question will be asked by those with coeliac disease 'what is the long-term future for me?' This chapter is not aimed at speculation; it looks at the here and now of chronic disease management and its implication for the future of those with coeliac disease and discusses the future direction of research.

CHRONIC DISEASE MANAGEMENT

There is (BSG, 2006; Department of Health, 2004a, 2004b) an acknowledged increase in the burden of chronic disease worldwide. It consumes a large proportion of health and social care resources. This is largely accounted for by increased attendance at the doctors and more inpatient days. Despite the chronicity of coeliac disease it rarely accounts for such a large drain on resources when followed up and managed effectively.

It is suggested (Milne, 2007) that the best care for people with chronic conditions is delivered when resources and services are integrated and focused on empowering the patient to provide effective self-care. After all, as acknowledged (Department of Health, 2004b), healthcare professionals will probably interact with people with chronic disease only for a few hours a year after which time, even with the best support services, patients are left to manage for themselves. With secondary care becoming more focused on being an acute care provider, there is an impetus to ensure that the service integration between primary and secondary care is robust – the principles being to take care closer to the patient and in the case of coeliac disease involving patients in their own care and encouraging self-management. This necessitates closer integration of care between primary and secondary care providers with the provision of education, training and agreed pathways of care using a multidisciplinary approach (BSG, 2006).

The Department of Health adopted and adapted a pyramid from Kaiser Permanente to illustrate how the needs of chronic disease patients differ (Figure 9.1).

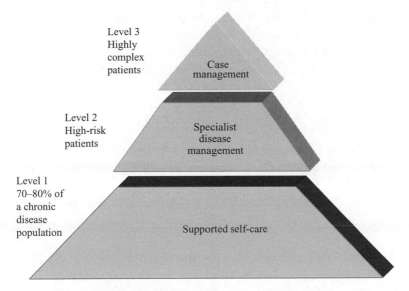

Level 3
Highly
complex
patients

Case
management

Level 2
High-risk
patients

Specialist
disease
management

Level 1
70–80% of
a chronic
disease
population

Supported self-care

Figure 9.1   Pyramid of care.

Most coeliac patients will sit at level one and much of the discussion in previous chapters has centred on the information, knowledge and support to self-manage, including expert patient programmes. Those at level two will inevitably be those who have difficulty adhering to their gluten free diet and need additional specialist input but can be managed following agreed protocols and pathways. Those at level three will be those with complex medical and social problems, which may mean that they have more than one chronic disease or medical condition requiring specialist input and a more holistic approach (Department of Health, 2004b). The success of a chronic disease management programme requires not only multidisciplinary team work but as acknowledged by the British Society of Gastroenterology (BSG, 2006), a greater overlap of specialist nursing support between primary and secondary care. This is therefore an ideal opportunity for appropriately trained nurses with a role in the management of coeliac patients to support service development, providing a quality specialist service that is appreciated by both patients and healthcare professionals alike. As political climates change so too do the drivers, targets and financial flows that support service development and nurses need to demonstrate an awareness of these factors throughout the planning process.

Activity

Look at the current political drivers; what might be their impact on ongoing services for coeliac patients? Consider both the positive and negative impacts. Current drivers will include practice-based commissioning, payment by results, but be aware that these might change.

The first step in chronic disease management is in being able to identify the population with that specific condition or conditions. Unlike chronic health conditions such as diabetes, chronic heart failure and chronic obstructive pulmonary disease, there are no National Service Frameworks (NSFs) or NICE guidance for coeliac disease and as a result no quality and outcomes frameworks (QOFs) to reward the collection of patient registers within primary care to ensure that they are able to identify the coeliac population to follow them up effectively. This means establishing alternative evidence-based service provision models.

Figure 9.2 shows an example for service provision developed by the author. A service level agreement (SLA) is in essence a contract between two service providers outlining the common understanding about the service to be provided, the priorities and the lines of accountability, the main purpose being to agree on the level of service.

In the example shown the SLA carries a financial benefit for primary care as the proposed provider, as they retain payment for the follow-up of each patient but there is also an agreed payment for the support of specialist gastroenterology services.

The model serves only as one example of what can be achieved with close interdisciplinary working.

SERVICE LEVEL AGREEMENT

Local Enhanced Service for the follow-up of patients with a confirmed diagnosis of coeliac disease

1.   **Service Aims**
       The management of coeliac disease is acknowledged as an increasing part of a gastroenterologist's workload. Recent prevalence studies suggest that 1% of the general UK population have positive coeliac serology.

       Coeliac disease as a chronic, permanent condition requires lifelong follow-up to avoid unnecessary morbidity including:
       • Growth retardation in childhood
       • Osteoporosis and/or Osteopenia
       • Development of autoimmune disorders
       • Anaemia
       • Malignancy
       • Neurological disease
       • Infertility
       • Chronic fatigue

       The British Society of Gastroenterology (BSG, 2002) and the Primary Care Society for Gastroenterology (PCSG, 2006) recommend annual follow-up for patients with uncomplicated, stable disease.

       The aim of this service would be to:
       • Enhance the continuity of care
       • Ensure that the service is timely and convenient to the patient
       • Facilitate chronic disease management within the most appropriate setting

       Patients with more complex needs that do not meet the service protocol would continue to be seen in secondary care by the specialist team.

2.   **Finance Details**

3.   **Criteria**
       The Local Enhanced Services Specification details the following criteria taken from the PCSG (2006) recommendations:

       • The practice creates a database of coeliac disease patients to facilitate recall and audit.
       • There is a template to record clinical data in a standardised way to facilitate audit and research.
       • There is a named person who has clinical and administrative responsibility for the service.
       The following criteria are considered in developing the management pathway.

       3.1 Annual Assessment
       The annual assessment should involve:
       • Assessment of and motivation towards, strict adherence to a gluten-free diet.
       • Ensuring appropriate prescription of gluten-free products as requested by patient.
       • Measurement of weight, height and body mass index.
       • Assessment of symptoms, including general well-being and bowel function.
       • Routine blood tests: haemoglobin, iron studies including ferritin, folate, serum albumin and alkaline phosphatase.
       • Assessment of any suspected nutritional deficiencies by checking blood levels of calcium, vitamin A, D, E and B12.
       • Osteoporosis risk assessment.

       3.2 Osteoporosis Assessment and Management
       • DEXA should be undertaken at diagnosis, at the menopause for women, at the age of 55 years for men, at any age if fracture occurs, where significant risk exists.
       • Advise regular physical activity, reducing smoking and alcohol consumption.
       • Advise on appropriate calcium intake. Consider supplementation if adequate dietary intake cannot be maintained (i.e. lactose intolerant)
       • Prescribe appropriate treatment if the patient is osteopenic/osteoporotic. Assess adherence to and side effects of any treatment.

Figure 9.2 Model – example of enhanced service agreement.

3.3 Management of Possible Splenic Atrophy
Splenic atrophy will occur to some degree in patients with coeliac disease. Patients should therefore be considered for:
- Vaccination against penumococcus and haemophilus influenzae type B.
- Vaccination against influenza.

3.4 Referral to the Gastroenterologist
Referral back to the specialist team should be considered if there is:
- Poor response to the gluten-free diet despite education and dietetic support
- Weight loss on a gluten-free diet
- Change in bowel habit, including blood in stools
- Unexplained abdominal pain
- Persistent unexplained abnormalities in blood results

Demonstration that the practice fulfils these criteria have been agreed at a practice meeting between a member of the specialist gastroenterology team and the named healthcare professional in the practice responsible for delivering the service.

DATE OF PRACTICE VISIT	NAME	SIGNATURE

4. **Accreditation**
Accreditation is based on fulfilment of the above criteria with further training and educational input from a member of the specialist gastroenterology team as required.

5. **Performance Monitoring Arrangements**
The aim of this Local Enhanced Service is to provide high quality, consistent follow-up care for patients with uncomplicated, stable coeliac disease. Under this service arrangement the practice is obliged to provide the PCT with annual data that demonstrates appropriate follow-up for all patients as a result of this service.

The practice should undertake an annual review of this service which should include:
- Clinical criteria as outlined by the specialist gastroenterology team
- Length of time and number of consultations required
- Any difficulties encountered running the service
- Patient feedback

The clinical information required will include:
- The number of patients with coeliac disease at the practice
- The number of patients followed up in the review period
- Percentage compliant with a gluten-free diet
- Nutritional status – including weight and body mass index
- Osteoporosis risk assessment

This document constitutes the agreement between the practice and the PCT in regards to the delivery of the agreed local enhanced service specifications.

Signed on behalf of the practice:

SIGNATURE	NAME	DATE

Signed on behalf of the PCT:

SIGNATURE	NAME	DATE

Figure 9.2 *(continued)*

FUTURE RESEARCH INTO COELIAC DISEASE

We know that gluten is a common ingredient in the diet and that even trace amounts of gluten will contaminate foods thought to be gluten free. Therefore, strict adherence to a gluten free diet can prove to be a significant challenge. If that challenge is 'life long' then it is understandable that research is increasingly becoming centred on finding a normal 'non-toxic' diet that will improve the quality of life for those individuals with coeliac disease and reduce the risk of secondary autoimmune disorders and gastrointestinal malignancies, the ultimate aim – a cure?

As was highlighted in the very first chapter outlining the history of the disease, even recent findings become confined to history as more is uncovered about the disease. In the last few years there has been huge progress into understanding just how coeliac disease is triggered with identification of the dominant wheat protein epitopes. This in turn has opened the door to the opportunity of finding ways to eliminate what we know to be the detrimental gluten peptides from the diet or to dull their immune stimulatory effects.

What follows are just a few examples of the areas of research and development that may eventually lead to a change in the management of these patients.

Oral supplementation with prolyl endopeptidases

Among the main dietary proteins gluten has a high glutamine and proline content which prevents proteolysis by gastric, pancreatic and brush border enzymes, resulting in the build-up of oligopeptides (a small number of amino acids linked together) that are toxic to patients with coeliac disease. The finding that one of the key T-cell stimulatory peptides in coeliac disease is resistant to breakdown by intestinal proteases has created interest in developing proline and glutamine-specific prolyl endopeptidases (PEPs) as a therapeutic agent with the ability to detoxify proteolytically resistant gluten epitopes before they reach the small intestine where gluten induces the inflammatory T-cell responses that lead to coeliac disease.

The use of non-human proteases for gluten detoxification was proposed as far back as the late 1950s (Kranik & Mohn, 1959) and a clinical trial in 1976 (Messer & Baume, 1976) was inconclusive. The problem with many of the PEP studies to date has been that they have been irreversibly inactivated by the pepsin and acid pH of the stomach and as a consequence have failed to degrade gluten before it reaches the small intestine. More recently, researchers (Stepniak *et al.*, 2006) have evaluated a PEP from *Aspergillus niger*, which works optimally between pH 4 and 5 but is stable at pH of 2, is completely resistant to digestion with pepsin and in this trial effectively degraded all tested T-cell stimulatory peptides in addition to intact gluten molecules. A further recent study (Gass *et al.*, 2007) has evaluated a combination therapy, consisting of two gastrically active enzymes one of which, *Sphingomonas capsulata*, again has an extended pH profile. These appear to show promising results to date, with evidence for the existence of other promising gastrically active glutenases in germinating cereals (Hartmann *et al.*, 2006). Understandably to be acceptable for treatment of a largely non-life-threatening disease for which a dietary alternative is available, any novel therapy has to be entirely safe, effective and cost neutral (Schuppan & Junker, 2007).

Transamidation of wheat flour

This novel approach has more recently been described (Gianfrani *et al.*, 2007). Gianfrani and colleagues (2007) started with the principle of oral prolyl endopeptidase therapy as a strategy, one not requiring full knowledge of the toxic sequence of gluten and from there they explored the potential of transglutaminase activity. They treated whole-wheat flour with a low-molecular-weight microbial transglutaminase (mTG) and lysine methyl ester. This caused a drastic reduction in the gliadin-specific interferon γ expression in gliadin-specific intestinal T-cell lines generated from the biopsy specimens of 12 adult patients with coeliac disease. In slightly simpler terms, they found that they were able to detoxify gluten by exploiting the same substrate specificity of transglutaminase that leads to more potent immunostimulatory gluten peptides via deamidation (Schuppan & Junker, 2007).

Microbial transglutaminase is already used widely by the food industry as a dough improver and for improving the texture of foods (Yokoyama *et al.*, 2004), which certainly makes it attractive to patients with coeliac disease given the current volume and texture of breads!

However, there are several issues that remain to be resolved (Schuppan & Junker, 2007). Amongst these are concerns as to just how complete transamidation of gluten peptides can be reliably achieved in flours by treatment with mTG and lysine methyl ester given that some patients react to even trace amounts of gluten. The practicality of large-scale production and cost of these flours is also a consideration; will these be made available on prescription? Another uncertainty is around the imprecise involvement of innate immunity in the pathogenesis of coeliac disease. Innate immunity appears to be independent of gluten deamidation, the peptides involved in innate immunity being different from those driving adaptive immunity. The pre-activation of the innate immune system may well decide how the adaptive immune system recognises gluten. Larger scale clinical trials will obviously be needed, with more sensitive measures such as cytokine expression in intestinal biopsies before and after challenge (Schuppan & Junker, 2007).

Genetically modified crops

When we first think of genetically modified (GM) crops, many may think back to the American agricultural company, Monsanto, whose focus on applying technology and innovation to improve the success of farming led to its ill-fated advertising campaign to introduce GM seeds to the European market. Coming at a time when consumers were anxious about the safety of foods following the bovine spongiform encephalitis (BSE) epidemic, it forced the European Union to impose an effective moratorium on GM crops in 1998, an imposition which the European commission is now planning to lift to allow only the first commercially grown genetically modified crops, namely maize and potato in British and European fields (Leake, 2007).

Known as biotechnology and using the technique of 'gene splicing' or 'recombinant DNA technology' (rDNA), scientists can add new genetic information to create a novel protein which creates new traits, such as resistance to disease and pests. The future could include famine relief using GM cereals as part of food aid and genetically modifying foods to contain certain vaccines. Although as yet uncertain it may in the same way be possible to generate cereals with absent or reduced immunogenicity and in the future be possible to create a strain of commercially useful crops and overcome all T-cell stimulatory sequences (Van Heel & West, 2006). However, the problem with trying to mutate the DNA that encodes toxic gluten sequences is that it has been estimated that there are around 50 immunodominant gluten epitopes that would have to be eliminated. Some varieties of ancient wheat appear to have fewer toxic T-cell sequences and these might be a better starting material for detoxification (Schuppan & Junker, 2007).

Environmentalists have expressed concerns over issues such as herbicide-tolerant plants themselves becoming invasive weeds with the herbicide tolerance then spreading to wild plants through cross-pollination, damaging biodiversity. Therefore, whatever the outcome it will be necessary for a good deal of positive research to reassure the public that GM crops actually are of benefit and not simply aimed at lining the pockets of multinational corporations.

Back to the future

Currently, without evidence of the long-term effects of some treatments it is difficult to assess their benefits when we already have a robust and safe, albeit burdensome, treatment for a non-life-threatening disease in the form of the gluten free diet. There is some evidence to suggest (Matysiak-Budnik *et al.*, 2007) that up to 10% of patients diagnosed with coeliac disease in childhood spontaneously recover a normal villous architecture after a prolonged period on a normal gluten-containing diet without any of the clinical or biological manifestations of coeliac disease. They do however retain immunological evidence of the disease, meaning that there is still the risk of relapse, and long-term follow-up remains essential. However, this apparent return to 'latency' as described in silent disease does raise some important questions regarding what factors promote that return?

There are still many questions left to answer, made more difficult by the absence of a good animal model of coeliac disease, that will allow studies to be undertaken into more novel therapeutics (Van Heel & West, 2006). Until then the mainstay of treatment for coeliac disease must remain adherence to a gluten free diet and the nurses' role in promoting and supporting that adherence remains of paramount importance. This necessitates an understanding of what it means to live with coeliac disease now, remembering that as our understanding of the disease increases and new interventions are established the disease itself changes to become in effect a 'new' disease.

HINTS AND TIPS

- Find out what the current drivers are for chronic disease management in your area. How can you influence the inclusion of coeliac disease in any developments to ensure that follow-up is maintained? What will be your role?
- Bearing in mind the sometimes dubious quality of available information, ensure that you can source reliable information on current research. Media sensationalism will often need to be followed by a more measured explanation and sometimes reassurance.

REFERENCES

British Society of Gastroenterology (2006) *Care of Patients with Gastrointestinal Disorders in the United Kingdom: A Strategy for the Future*. BSG, London.

Department of Health (2004a) *Improving Chronic Disease Management*. Department of Health, London.

Department of Health (2004b) *Chronic Disease Management: A Compendium of Information*. http://www.natpact.nhs.uk/uploads/Chronic%20Care%20Compendium.pdf. Accessed 2 October 2007.

Gass, J., Bethune, M.T., Siegel, M., Spencer, A. & Khosla, C. (2007) Combination enzyme therapy for gastric digestion of dietary gluten in patients with coeliac sprue. *Gastroenterology* 133(2):472–480.

Gianfrani, C., Siciliano, R., Facchiano, A., Camarca, A., Mazzeo, M., Constantini, S., Salvati, V., Maurano, F., Mazzarella, G., Iaquinto, G., Bergamo, P. & Rossi, M. (2007) Transamidation of wheat flour inhibits the response to gliadin of intestinal T cells in coeliac disease. *Gastroenterology* 133:780–789.

Hartmann, P., Koehler, P. & Wieser, H. (2006) Rapid degradation of gliadin peptides toxic for coeliac disease patients by proteases from germinating cereals. *Journal of Cereal Science* 44:368–371.

Kranik, H.G. & Mohn, G. (1959) Further investigations on the toxic effect of wheat flour in coeliac disease: Effect of enzymatic by products of gliadin. *Helvetica Paediatrica Acta* 14:124–140.

Leake, J. (2007) Europe set to lift ban on genetically modified crops. *The Times* [on line], July 1st. http://www.timesonline.co.uk/tol/news/uk/science/article2011074.ece. Accessed 15 October 2007.

Matysiak-Budnick, T., Malamut, G., Patey-Mariaud de Serre, N., Grosdidier, E., Seguier, S., Brousse, N., Caillat-Zucman, S., Cerf-Bensussan, N., Schmitz, J. & Cellier, C. (2007) Long-term follow-up of 61 patients diagnosed in childhood: Evolution toward latency is possible on a normal diet. *Gut* 56:1379–1386.

Messer, M. & Baume, P.E. (1976) Oral papain in Gluten intolerance. *The Lancet* 2:1022.

Milne, C. (2007) *Chronic Disease Management*. http://www.nhsconfed.org/specialist/specialist-1658.cfm. Accessed 1 October 2007.

Schuppan, D. & Junker, Y. (2007) Turning swords into plowshares: Transglutaminase to detoxify gluten (Editorial). *Gastroenterology* 133:1025–1038.

Stepniak, D., Spaenij-Dekking, L., Mitea, C., Moester, M., DeRu, A., Baak-Pablo, R., Van Veelen, P., Edens, L. & Koning, F. (2006) Highly efficient gluten degradation with a newly identified prolyl endoprotease: Implications for coeliac disease. *American Journal of Physiology: Gastrointestinal and Liver Physiology* 291:G621–G629.

Van Heel, D. & West, J. (2006) Recent advances in coeliac disease. *Gut* 55:1037–1046.

Yokoyama, K., Nio, N. & Kikuchi, Y. (2004) Properties and applications of microbial transglutaminase. *Applied Microbiological Biotechnology* 64:447–454.

Chapter 10
Patients' Stories

It would only be fitting that the final word in a book on the nursing care and management of patients with coeliac disease should be given by those with the disease. Most of the inspiration for this book has come from those that I have cared for over the years in specialist practice. I have only to mention my interest to find that I am sitting next to managers in meetings with coeliac disease, in far-flung corners of the globe holidaying with coeliac patients or even finding that my daughters' friends have the disease. If we look for it and are aware of it, we find that it surrounds us. Yet it still remains underdiagnosed and largely unrecognised as a chronic disease but it can have a huge impact on the lives of those that it touches. As nurses we can help minimise that impact.

The stories that conclude this book are true stories written by patients, patients who are truly 'engaged' in their own care and therefore empowered to self-manage. These skills only come with the education, information and ongoing support that allow confidence to flourish and their stories are a testimony to the journey of many.

As Oscar Wilde said in *The Importance of Being Ernest* (Wilde, 1898):

> There is only one thing in the world worse than being talked about, and that is not being talked about.

Hence this book.

ALAN'S STORY

I am a 43-year-old male who was diagnosed with coeliac disease in 2006. It has taken me a little while to get to this point; however, I am now happily putting on weight, getting fitter and looking forward to the future. I have written briefly about my experiences in the hope that it will help others.

Symptoms and consequences

With the benefit of hindsight, I can see how the effects of coeliac have impacted on my life; however, my first obvious symptom was that of anaemia. This was picked up when I went to give blood in 2002 and was turned away as my iron levels were too low. This was perhaps the reason why I always felt tired; however, my job as a project manager involved long hours, so I expected tiredness to come with the job.

The anaemia was resolved with a course of iron tablets from the doctor and left at that. What I did not realise at the time was that I had started to compensate the tiredness by doing less. The crunch came when I was offered a project that involved a regular daily commute from home to the client site, about an hour and a half drive each way. Pretty soon I was starting to struggle. When I realised that I could not cope with the demands of this project I tried to get moved off the project; it did not help that the company I worked for thought that 16 h days were a good thing? With no medical reason and little support from my employer I began to wonder if I was suffering from burnout. Clearly to continue on this project would be suicidal and with the long hours and long-distance commuting I decided to down shift and see if that helped. I got a part-time job at a local school working just 25 h, hoping that a career change would make a difference. Talking to former colleagues, I had a lucky escape, at the time of writing four of the project team members are off sick with stress.

Despite this change, I continued to feel tired; I would come home, walk the dogs, and then fall asleep on the sofa, all before 6 pm. I seemed to pick up every bug at the school and suffered from aches and pains and lack of concentration. It seemed like

I had a season ticket at the doctors, and every time I went I would be told that there were no obvious reason, which would add to my frustration.

Eventually my wife, who by this time was sure I was really not well, escorted me to the doctors. Unbeknown to me, my wife had spoken to my mother who had said I had been very ill as a baby and the doctors had said that they thought I was a 'coeliac baby' and that I would grow out of the problem. No formal testing was done.

At the doctors we saw a locum who my wife badgered into doing a test for coeliac disease.

Diagnosis

The blood test came back positive and I was told that I would have to have some more tests but would need to go on to a gluten-free diet. At this point, I was happy to try anything. I went home and did some research about gluten-free (GF) diets. I had not been told at this point to stay on food with gluten in it until I had actually had the endoscope test, so I started on my GF diet. I started to feel better after a few weeks and after a couple of months I started to feel much better. Then came the letter with the hospital appointment, which said I was not supposed to go onto a GF diet until I had the endoscope test. My test was in January 2006, so I had to go back on the gluten over the Christmas of 2005; I consoled myself by enjoying what was to be my last chance to drink Guinness.

When it came to my test I was given two choices, I could have a sedative or a throat spray prior to the endoscope test, although I had the impression that if I had the sedative I would be guilty of using up unnecessary hospital resources and be a bit of a pansy in the process. So, being a bloke I opted for the throat spray. What they do not tell you until after the first squirt is that the throat spray tastes worse than you can imagine, and you have got another squirt coming.

Despite the rising panic after looking at what seemed to be a large plastic snake with two glowing eyes on the table next to me, the actual experience was fairly painless. The large boa constrictor being stuffed down your throat felt a little uncomfortable and was clearly something you would not want to do at home, but was bearable for the short duration of the test. The only unpleasant bit was when the consultant asked for some pictures to be taken as the endoscope was being removed with the result that it was unceremoniously stuffed back down my throat, which resulted in a brief moment of discomfort and the urge to throw up. On the positive side you get a nice nurse to hold your hand during the proceedings!

So, finally on the 27th January 2006, I get the result confirmed; I have coeliac disease and have to go on GF diet.

I had to have two further tests, one a DEXA scan to see if your bones have been weakened by lack of calcium and the other a series of X-rays of your insides to make sure you do not have any signs of bowel cancer. A word of advice here is not to watch Alien shortly before the X-ray and not to worry too much about what you see on the screen during the procedure.

In addition to the above tests, I had a regular check-up during my first year to make sure that I was managing well and sticking to the diet and thereafter get an annual check-up to make sure everything is going well.

Getting to grips with the diet

The GF diet sounds like it should be easy; however, there are problems with cross-contamination and mistakenly eating something because you did not expect it to have gluten in. Over the last couple of years, I have had a couple of problems; one through eating a takeaway that was supposed to be safe and secondly eating too much food with modified wheat starch in it (Codex standard!). I think I have got the diet cracked now; if in doubt do not eat it and always have food with you because it can be very hard to get a GF meal when you are out.

One of the essential requirements of having coeliac disease is the ability to get certain foods on prescription; although a lot of food is available commercially it is often very expensive and can require a visit to several supermarkets in order to complete the weekly shop and then sometimes you can discover that the supermarket is out of stock. Being able to get food on prescription ensures that you are able to get the food that you need when you need it. Imagine how difficult it would be to stick to the diet if you went to three different shops and still be unable to get the bread you need to make sandwiches.

Support and advice

One thing I have found is that it helps to talk to other people in the same position, especially if you have just been diagnosed. Quite often people are told things at the hospital but it does not always sink in at the time and it is much easier to ask questions with someone else who has had the same experience and also has much more time to talk about cross-contamination, shopping, eating out and avoiding unexpected foods.

A key source of information is Coeliac U.K., which is the charity that supports people with coeliac disease and dermatitis herpetiformis (DH). The charity has a number of local support groups that are run by members, and provides help and guidance to people who are diagnosed with coeliac disease and DH.

I went to our local support group annual general meeting with my wife and came out as the group organisers. My wife and I have been running the group for 6 months and have organised a number of events like coffee mornings, GF fish and chip evenings and by far the largest a GF food fair. This took 3 months to organise and much hard work by my wife who spent hours on the phone after work talking to suppliers and organising press coverage, advertising and radio interviews for the event. In the end, we had nearly 1400 people from a wide area. We have had lots of positive feedback from everyone who took part and from numerous people who attended.

I always find that when I talk to someone at an event I always learn something new, whether it is a type of food that I can now eat or benefiting from hearing someone else's experience. It is very easy to feel isolated on a GF diet, so it is always worthwhile to talk to someone else in the same position.

The future

I have been on my GF diet for nearly 2 years now and feel pretty confident about it. My fitness has improved, as well as my stamina. I started to put on weight after the first 6 months of the diet, but now I am doing more exercise and my weight has stabilised at a respectable amount. My brain is working properly and I can actually remember things for more than 2 min now.

I have been working as an administrator for the last year for the local authority and am now starting to take on more responsibility as I have the energy for bigger and better things. I have just recently been seconded to a large transformation project with lots more opportunities.

Being ill with coeliac disease has had a major impact on my earnings and eaten away all of my savings. Getting back on my feet has been a bit of a struggle but now I feel that my life is going in the right direction. I am extremely grateful for all the help I have had from the specialist staff at the hospital, dietitians, the coeliac support group and especially my wife. I think it would have taken me a lot longer to get to this position. (I still miss my Guinness though!)

ZOE'S STORY

Initial symptoms

In December 2005, I went to the local GP complaining of per-sistent headaches, double vision, achy eyes and was concerned that occasionally when speaking my words would become muddled. I really struggled at work and remember having many moments in the toilets feeling exhausted and generally unwell.

I was very surprised when the GP referred me to see the neurologist at Hereford Hospital. I really believed that I was wasting the neurologist's time, as I thought that maybe I just needed a pair of glasses! After the examination by the neurologist, I was horrified to hear that there were two outcomes that he suspected were the cause of my headaches and muddled speech. One was a tumour on the cerebellum and the other was fluid on the brain. I was horrified! I was sent for a brain scan ASAP. To my relief they came back negative; the neurologist was baffled! I then had a lumbar puncture and many bloods taken. The neurologist had noticed that my eyes were making involuntary movements. This was diagnosed as oscillopsia, but the specialists and doctors were unsure what was causing this movement.

Coeliac disease

After a painful few months of worry and tests, one of the bloods came back showing that I had coeliac disease (lumbar puncture normal). This completely threw me, as I was well aware of what this disease was. Two of my aunties were coeliac, and they had bowel symptoms. After three endoscopies, it was definitely confirmed that I had coeliac disease. At the time the specialists saw no link between my symptoms and the diagnosis. I was also sent for a bone scan to see if I had osteoporosis; the results were returned as entirely normal.

The neurologist at Hereford referred me to see a consultant neuro-ophthalmic surgeon in Birmingham. After yet another examination he was unable to say whether or not it was linked to coeliac. Unfortunately, my eyes seemed to be getting worse, although I had been on a strict GF diet.

I became increasingly worried and was desperate for answers. I was very concerned about my eyes, and it was so emotionally difficult, knowing that none of the specialists could give me a diagnosis.

After this appointment and with still no answers, I decided to seek help from a homoeopath. I spent an increasingly huge amount of money and tried many different potions. (None of these seemed to have worked.)

I had to have time off work due to my involuntary eye movements; they caused me to feel extremely sick and as I was trying to keep my eyes focused I encountered many headaches and felt physically drained.

I was then referred to a professor at Leicester Royal Infirmary, who is a neuro-ophthalmic surgeon. She was unsure about whether I had coeliac disease or cerebella ataxia or spinal cerebellar ataxia. I had no idea about these medical conditions, and at the time I was 3 months' pregnant (A VERY STRESSFUL TIME!)

I researched these conditions on the internet; they were very alarming to read. I went to speak to my GP about them; unfortunately, he was very supportive but unable to shed any light on the topic of the illnesses.

I decided to try and put everything to the back of my mind and concentrate on my pregnancy. I am due to go back to Leicester Hospital for yet more tests!

I am still committed to maintaining my GF diet in the hope that one day my eye movements will come back to normal. I am lucky to live in Wales as prescriptions are free, so I can stock up on lots of GF foods. It is amazing to see the improvement in taste and variety in GF foods over the last 18 months!! (Thank God!).

JEAN'S STORY

Initial symptoms

When I was in my twenties (and I am now 70), I suffered with awful bouts of diarrhoea and after a number of admissions to hospital I was diagnosed with Crohn's disease. Despite taking tablets, I continued to suffer spates of diarrhoea and abdominal pain so severe that I could not get on a bus into town without being incontinent. I was always worn out and my weight was less than six stone; I could have some good spells but they were not many, and in the end my marriage broke down, leaving me with two small children to bring up.

A nervous disposition

At this time the diarrhoea was worse but the doctor said that they did not think I had Crohn's at all but irritable bowel syndrome and that the diarrhoea was because I had a nervous disposition made worse by the break-up of my marriage.

Eventually, I remarried at 34 and one night I was really doubled up with pain and the doctor was called out and they got me into hospital for an exploratory operation. They found some inflammation but said that it was not Crohn's but irritable bowel. I had a third child and continued to suffer with bouts of diarrhoea, pain and exhaustion. My husband kept telling me to pull myself together and that I was making the diarrhoea worse by worrying. I felt ashamed of myself. I felt that I was not a woman; I had lost interest in sex and did not want anyone to touch me. I felt so dirty and needed to have constant baths.

A diagnosis at last

About 3 or 4 years after the exploratory operation I went to Benidorm with my sisters for a short break. For the whole week I had diarrhoea from morning to night; it did not matter what I ate. I was really unwell and my sisters said, this is really silly you must go back to see the doctor; this cannot go on.

So, when I got back I went to see Dr Johnson. She was really lovely; she sent me for some tests; and within 10 days I had a diagnosis of coeliac disease. It was wonderful: firstly, I had been frightened that I had something like cancer, as there was a lot of cases of cancer in my family and my mother died of stomach cancer; and secondly, it was great to know that I was not a lunatic! I started on the diet – which was really difficult then because there was not much around and there was not any follow-up or support, but within months I felt so much better. I had loads of energy, my skin was better and I started to put on weight. I was happier than I had ever been. I was working and running youth clubs; it was great.

The slippery slope

Then my husband suffered a heart attack and things got difficult. I suppose I was trying to hold down two jobs, look after my husband and the children; my eldest daughter was living with us with her baby as well and my diet went to the wall.

I also had problems with chest pain and was diagnosed with angina. Eventually, I started to feel ill again because obviously I was not sticking to my diet and eventually went back down to the hospital about 7 years ago. It has not been easy because there have been a lot of domestic issues; the family moaned at the expense of buying 'special' food just for me. I think that when you tell someone that you have an 'allergy' which is what it is really, then they do not realise the importance of it. They think of it like they would hives. They say, oh go on 'a little bit won't hurt you' but as the dietitian said a little bit will. As the nurses say I must tell them it is a disease. It is getting easier in fact; my children and my husband now come home with the odd 'GF' treat. I still sometimes struggle especially if I am eating out and I order something that I think is gluten free and then find that there is something in it that perhaps is not. I sometimes still get black looks from the family when I am pushing food round the plate, examining it and then I find myself using my weight as an excuse for not eating it rather than mentioning the coeliac disease. My life is definitely getting better, but I could not have stuck at it without the support and patience of the dietitians and nurses. I am now very strict with myself because I do not want to be a sick old lady and I have a sick husband and my grandchildren to look after.

I know that doctors are only human and they did sympathise with me, but I did not want sympathy. I just wanted practical advice so that I could live my life, perhaps a little sooner?

MRS A'S STORY

Early recollections

I was born in the early 1950s. I was diagnosed at 15 months as having coeliac disease. Not very much appeared to be known at the time, at this time, about what I could and could not eat – only that fruit was allowed and bread had to be specially made for me at home. Fruit, however, was scarce as food was still rationed following the end of the Second World War. My family exchanged coupons with friends so that I could have sufficient fruit for my diet. My earliest recollections of being on a different diet was going to friends' birthday parties with my own food.

As research into the condition progressed, my family doctor kept my parents informed of different foods that I was allowed to eat. There was no coeliac society then to given guidance about the condition. I was a pre-school child before the all clear came, allowing me to eat potatoes – still my favourite vegetable.

Cured

The theory in the 1960s was that once a person with coeliac disease had become a teenager they no longer had the allergy. Consequently, I was gradually weaned off the diet and started to eat 'normal' foods. I went to guide camps and, after studying for 'A' levels, went to a teacher training college, living away from home for 3 years. I went on holidays abroad, married and settled into my own home. I would have occasional bouts of diarrhoea but I would always resort to eating bananas until it passed. Unknown to me at the time, this was considered the correct thing to do.

Pregnancy

After a year of marriage, I became pregnant. The pregnancy progressed well with the only difference between me and other pregnant women being that I only put on 10 lb in weight during the pregnancy. Unfortunately, my waters broke two and a half weeks before the due date and I had to have an emergency caesarean section. My daughter was perfectly formed and weighed in at 6 lb 9 oz. However, after a few weeks I started to have constant diarrhoea and was admitted to hospital when my daughter was nine and a half weeks old. It was in the hospital that I was given a biopsy test and told that I had to back on a GF diet for the rest of my life, as the villi in my small intestine were found to be completely flat. The specialist was not sure whether it had been my pregnancy, the birth or the caesarean section which caused the coeliac condition to recur.

Better support

I contacted the coeliac society and was sent information about a GF diet and about the research that was going on at the time into the condition. I obtained a copy of the GF food and drink directory and became a member of the coeliac society. Ever since then I have kept strictly to the diet and find that I can live a more or less normal life.

My second pregnancy progressed as normal. I put on two stones in weight and my second child was born a week late in a normal delivery.

About 7 years ago, after the menopause finished; I was sent for a DEXA scan to measure my bone density. It was found that I had some bone thinning and I was put on a weekly tablet to improve my bone density. This, I understand, has improved but I have a repeat scan every 2–3 years.

Putting on the Ritz

I have found that since I was a teenager many more foods have become available to suit the diet, making it much easier to cope as there is now more choice, although some items are very expensive. Since then also, however, a number of items for the diet have become available on prescription, making them more affordable. Health food shops and supermarkets have now begun to stock and increasingly wide range of products which has made catering for the family, special occasions and holidays much easier to manage. More people are now aware of the allergy and eating out in restaurants, cafes and hotels is much easier than it used to be. I am looking forward to going the Ritz Hotel in London in a few weeks, time as my family is treating me to tea – gluten free of course.

REFERENCE

Wilde, O. (1898) *The Importance of Being Ernest.* http://www.gutenberg.org/etext/844. Accessed 25 October 2007 (ebooks).

Glossary

Acute: In medicine meaning having a rapid onset and a short course.

Adaptive immunity: The adaptive immune system acts as a second line of defence and also affords protection against re-exposure to the same pathogen.

Aetiology (etiology): From the Greek 'giving a reason to' is the study of causation.

Algorithm: A predetermined list of well-defined instructions for accomplishing a stated task, proceeding through an explicit series of consecutive points to an end point.

Allele: One member of a pair or sequence of genes that occupies a specific position on a specific chromosome.

Anaemia: From the Greek 'without blood' is a deficiency of red blood cells and/or haemoglobin.

Antibody: Any of a range of proteins normally present in the body or produced in response to an antigen which it neutralises, producing an immune response.

Antigen: A molecule that stimulates an immune response.

Arthropathy: A disease or abnormality of a joint.

Assay: The purity of a substance or the amount or activity of any particular constituent of a mixture.

Autoimmune hepatitis: A disease in which the body's immune system attacks liver cells, causing the liver to become inflamed.

Autoimmunity: It is the failure of an organism to recognise its own constituent parts as 'self' resulting in an immune response against its own cells and tissues.

Avenin: It is the protein found in oats.

Cachexia: Severe weight loss, anorexia and general debility seen in chronic disease including cancers. Cachetic patients exhibit signs of malnutrition, including muscle wasting.

Carbohydrates: A compound consisting of carbon, hydrogen and oxygen. Major source of energy in the diet, includes sugars, starches and cellulose.

Cellulitis: A common bacterial infection of the lower layers of skin (dermis) and the subcutaneous tissues.

Cerebellar ataxia: A non-specific clinical manifestation implying dysfunction of parts of the nervous system in the part of the brain (cerebellum) that coordinates sensory perception and motor output.

Chronic: In medicine meaning having a slow onset and a long duration or frequent recurrence.

Chyme: A liquid resulting from the mechanical and chemical breakdown of a food bolus in the stomach consisting of partially digested food, water, hydrochloric acid and digestive enzymes.

Codex Alimentarius: Internationally recognised standards, codes of conduct and guidelines relating to food.

Collagenous colitis: It is a subtype of microscopic colitis with a peak incidence in the fifth decade of life, affecting women more than men. Presenting with non-bloody watery diarrhoea, normal colonoscopy but microscopically showing a distinctive thickening of subepithelial collagen.

Concomitant: Occurring or existing concurrently.

Cutaneous: Of, relating or affecting, the skin.

Cystic fibrosis: It is a hereditary disease affecting mainly the lungs and digestive system, causing progressive life-shortening disability.

Cytokines: Non-antibody proteins released by a cell population on contact with a specific antigen and acting as intercellular mediators, as in the generation of an immune response.

Deamidate: To remove the amide group from a compound.

Demographics: Refers to certain population characteristics used in government, marketing or opinion research.

DEXA: Dual-energy X-ray absorptiometry.

Emaciation: To make or become extremely thin.

Endocarditis: Inflammation of the inner lining of the heart (endocardium), caused by a bacterial infection.

Endomysium: Meaning within the muscle.

Enterocytes: A form of epithelial cell of the inner layer of the tissue lining the small and large intestine.

Enteropathy: Refers to any pathology of the intestine, gluten-sensitive enteropathy being another name for coeliac disease.

Enzymes: Proteins that accelerate chemical reactions.

Epithelium: Tissue composed of a layer of cells, lining the skin and the inside cavities of bodies.

Epitope: The part of a macromolecule that is recognised by the immune system, specifically by antibodies, B cells or T cells.

Erythrocyte: Red blood cell.

Exocrine: Secretion of enzymes into ducts as opposed to the secretion of hormones directly into the blood stream as in endocrine.

Fibroblasts: Maintain the structural integrity of connective tissue.

Flow cytometric immunophenotyping: A tool used in the diagnosis, classification, staging and monitoring of haematological cancers. It measures the percentages of specific lymphocytes amongst the total numbers of lymphocytes.

Folate: A water-soluble vitamin not stored by the body and therefore needed as part of the daily dietary intake.

Genetically modified: Modified organisms that have had their DNA altered through genetic engineering.

Genotype: The genetic constitution of an organism or a group of organisms.

Giardiasis: An intestinal infection caused by the microscopic parasite *Giardia lamblia*.

Gliadin: Any of several simple proteins derived from wheat, barley or rye gluten, capable of inducing a toxic response among individuals who lack the enzyme necessary for its digestion.

Gluten: A mixture of plant proteins occurring in cereal grains, wheat, barley and rye used as an adhesive.

Haemochromatosis: A hereditary disease characterised by the inappropriate metabolism of dietary iron causing iron overload and the accumulation of iron in organs such as the heart and liver.

Heterogeneity: The condition or state of being different in kind or nature.

Histopathology: The microscopic study of abnormal tissue and organs at their cellular level.

Hordein: The starchy matter contained in barley.

Hormone: From the Greek 'to set in motion', is a chemical messenger that carries a signal from one cell (or group of cells) to another.

Howell-jolly body: A spherical particle often observed in the stroma of a red blood cell, especially after a splenectomy.

Hypokalemia: A condition in which the body fails to retain sufficient potassium to maintain health, a potentially fatal condition.

Hypothyroidism: An abnormality of the thyroid gland characterised by insufficient production of thyroid hormone.

Idiopathic: Of, relating to, or designating a disease with no known cause.

Immunofluorescence: The use of antibodies chemically linked to a fluorescent dye to identify or quantify antigens in a tissue sample.

Immunoglobulin: A class of proteins produced in lymph tissue in vertebrates, which function as antibodies in the immune response.

Immunology: The branch of biomedicine concerned with the structure and function of the immune system and innate and acquired immunity, the body's distinction of self from non-self.

Immunopathogenesis: The process of development of a disease involving an immune response or the effects of an immune reaction.

Immunosuppressants: Refers to a group of drugs used to inhibit or prevent activity of the immune system.

Innate immunity: The innate immune system is our first line of defence against invading organisms.

Kamut: A type of wheat only registered as a plant variety in 1990.

Lacteal: An intestinal lymph-carrying vessel.

Lactose: A disaccharide making up around 8% of the solids found in milk.

Lamina propria: A thin layer of loose connective tissue lying beneath the epithelium which together with the epithelium constitutes the mucosa.

Latent: Present or potential but not evident or active, in a dormant or inactive phase.

Lymphocytes: Type of white blood cell with an integral role in the body's defences.

Lymphocytic colitis: A subtype of microscopic colitis, a rare condition characterised by chronic non-bloody watery diarrhoea. Normal macroscopic appearances but mucosal biopsy reveals an accumulation of lymphocytes in the epithelium and lamina propria.

Macrophages: From the Greek meaning 'big eater' their role is to engulf and then digest cellular debris and pathogens and to stimulate lymphocytes and other immune cells to respond to the pathogen.

Malabsorption: It is a state arising from an abnormality in the digestion or absorption of food in the gastrointestinal tract.

Mast cells: Cells found in connective tissue that releases substances such as heparin and histamine in response to injury or inflammation of bodily tissues.

Mesolithic: Of or relating to the cultural period of the Stone Age before the Neolithic periods marked by the emergence of stone tools and weapons and by changes in the nature of human settlement.

Microbe (micro-organism): An organism that is too small to be seen by the human eye.

Morphology: The study of the form or shape of an organism or part of an organism.

National Service Frameworks (NSFs): Policies set by the National Health Service in the United Kingdom to define standards of care for major medical issues such as cancer, coronary heart disease, mental health and diabetes and for some key patient groups including children and older people.

Neolithic: Also known as the New Stone Age, marked by the beginning of farming, the domestication of animals and the emergence of crafts such as pottery.

Neural tube defect: Normally, in human embryos, the closure of the neural tube occurs around the 30th day after fertilisation. However, if something interferes and the tube fails to close properly, a defect will occur (e.g. spina bifida).

Neuroendocrine: A specialised group of nerve cells that produce hormones.

Neuropathy: A disease or abnormality of the nervous system.

Neutrophils: The most abundant of the white blood cells, playing an integral part in the immune system.

NICE: National Institute of Clinical Excellence is an independent organisation responsible for providing national guidance on promoting good health and preventing and treating ill health.

Non-Hodgkin's lymphoma: It describes a group of cancers arising from lymphocytes of which gluten-sensitive enteropathy-associated T-cell lymphoma or EATL is one type.

Osteomyelitis: An acute or chronic infection of the bone and bone marrow.

Osteopenia: A bone disease in which there is a reduction in bone mass, less severe than that in osteoporosis. It is caused by the resorption of bone at a rate that exceeds bone synthesis (production).

Osteoporosis: A bone disease in which there is a decrease in bone mass and density, resulting in a high risk of fractures and bone deformities.

Otitis media: Inflammation of the middle ear.

Panacea: In medicine meaning a 'cure all'.

Pancreatic exocrine insufficiency: It is the inability to properly digest food due to the progressive loss of pancreatic cells leading to a lack of digestive enzymes.

Pancreolauryl test: A test of pancreatic function based on the specific splitting by pancreatic esterase of orally administered fluorescein dilaurate with a standard meal.

Papulovesicles: Small inflamed elevations of skin (papules) that become blisters.

Pathogen: Something that causes disease or illness to its host.

Pathogenesis: The development of a disease or disease-inducing condition.

Pathologic: Relating to or caused by disease.

Pericarditis: Inflammation of the pericardium, the fibrous sac surrounding the heart.

Peristalsis: The wave-like muscular contractions of the intestine that propel the contents onward by alternate contraction and relaxation.

Peritonitis: Inflammation of the peritoneum which is the serous membrane lining part of the abdominal cavity.

Phosphate: A salt of phosphoric acid.

Pneumococcus: A Gram-positive bacteria, major cause of pneumonia.

Primary biliary cirrhosis: Inflammation and loss of architecture in the liver as a result of chronic bile retention after obstruction or infection of the major extra/intrahepatic bile ducts.

Primary sclerosing cholangitis: A chronic liver disease characterised by inflammation, destruction and fibrosis of the intra and extrahepatic bile ducts that leading to cirrhosis of the liver.

Probiotics: These are bacterial or yeast cultures that are intended to assist the body's naturally occurring gut flora to re-establish themselves.

Prognosis: A prediction of the probable course and outcome of a disease.

Prolamine: A group of plant storage proteins with a high proline content found in the seeds of cereal grains.

Protein: It is made up of long chains of amino acids. Fundamental component of all living cells (enzymes, hormones and antibodies) as such essential in the diet for tissue growth and repair.

Protocol: A set of guidelines or rules that help in governing a process or procedure.

Pruritis: Intense itching, normally of undamaged skin.

Purkinje cells: These are a class of neuron located in the cerebellar cortex. They are named after their discoverer, Czechoslovakian anatomist Jan Evangelista Purkyně.

Quality and outcomes framework (QOF): It is the annual reward and incentive programme detailing GP practice achievement results.

Recombinant: A new entity such as a gene, protein or cell that results from genetic recombination.

Refractory: Resistant to treatment.

Reticulin: It is a histological term used to describe a type of structural fibre composed of type III collagen.

Screening: A systematic examination and assessment for the early detection of disease.

Secalin: A protein found in the grain rye.

Septic arthritis: An infection in the joint (synovial) fluid and joint tissues, usually reaching the joints through the blood stream.

Service level agreement (SLA): It is the part of a service contract where the level of service is formally defined.

Silent: Producing no detectable signs or symptoms.

Spelt: A species of wheat.

Sphincter: A circular muscle that normally maintains constriction of a natural body orifice, relaxing as required by normal physiological functioning.

Spina bifida: Partial closure of the embryonic neural tube results in an incompletely formed spinal cord; the vertebrae of the spine overlying the open portion of the spinal cord do not fully form and remain unfused and open.

Steatorrhoea: Abnormally high amounts of fat in the faeces which are frothy and foul smelling and floating; a symptom of disorders of fat metabolism and malabsorption.

Syndrome: An abnormal condition or disease diagnosed by a recognised group of signs and symptoms.

Titre: It is the unit in which the analytical detection of a substance is expressed, as a result of titration, a common laboratory method of chemical analysis.

Transamidation: The transfer of NH_2 from an amide moiety (e.g. from glutamine) to another molecule.

Transitional care: Refers to the actions of healthcare providers designed to ensure the coordination and continuity of healthcare during 'transition' from one care setting or care practitioner to another as an individual's needs change over the course of an illness or condition.

Tropical sprue: A chronic disorder that also occurs in non-tropical forms and in both children and adults. Characterised by failure to observe nutrients, symptoms include foul-smelling diarrhoea and emaciation.

Villi: Comes from the Latin 'shaggy hair' refers to the fine hair-like projections from the mucus membrane of the small intestine (plural of villous).

Villous atrophy: A decrease in the size of the villi as a result of injury/disease.

Index